THE STRUGGLE
FOR PUBLIC HEALTH

THE STRUGGLE FOR PUBLIC HEALTH

Seven People Who Saved the Lives of Millions
and Transformed the Way We Live

FRED C. PAMPEL

JOHNS HOPKINS UNIVERSITY PRESS | BALTIMORE

© 2024 Johns Hopkins University Press
All rights reserved. Published 2024
Printed in the United States of America on acid-free paper
9 8 7 6 5 4 3 2 1

Johns Hopkins University Press
2715 North Charles Street
Baltimore, Maryland 21218
www.press.jhu.edu

Library of Congress Cataloging-in-Publication Data is available.

A catalog record for this book is available from the British Library.

ISBN 978-1-4214-4793-3 (hardcover)
ISBN 978-1-4214-4794-0 (ebook)

*Special discounts are available for bulk purchases of this book. For more information,
please contact Special Sales at specialsales@jh.edu.*

CONTENTS

Introduction

Beginning in the late eighteenth century, for the first time in human history, the scourge of deadly infectious diseases began to permanently recede. In earlier centuries, cycles of plague, epidemics, and disease, often caused or accompanied by war, drought, and famine, kept the population in check and made life miserable for most everyone. In ancient Rome, the height of civilization at the time, a newborn could expect to live only twenty to thirty years on average.[1] The Middle Ages brought little improvement. Most deaths continued to occur soon after birth or in childhood, but adults remained at risk for cholera, influenza, typhus, smallpox, measles, and tuberculosis. Even after the Renaissance, when Europeans began to grow richer and learn more about disease, epidemics remained frighteningly common. The Great Plague of London in 1665–1666, for example, killed as many as one hundred thousand people, about 15 percent of the population.[2] King Charles II and the wealthy fled the city to avoid the plague, but most had to stay and accept that they could die at any time.

No wonder the seventeenth-century philosopher Thomas Hobbes called human life nasty, brutish, and short.

Progress against these diseases began in England in the late 1700s and picked up speed through the 1800s. The data on deaths and the specific causes are quite limited, but figures from roughly 1851 to 1900 illustrate the remarkable transformation.[3] Death rates from respiratory tuberculosis dropped by 49 percent, typhus by 79 percent, scarlet fever by 80 percent, smallpox by 94 percent, whooping cough by 16 percent, and diarrhea, dysentery, and cholera by 28 percent.

Perhaps surprisingly, the decline in deaths from communicable diseases appears to have begun well before the discovery of most vaccines and effective medical treatments. Trends in tuberculosis illustrate this claim. The steady downward trend in deaths from the disease dates back to at least 1851, most likely even earlier. Yet, effective treatment came much later. The tubercle bacillus was not identified until 1882, chemotherapy for tuberculosis was introduced in 1947, and substantial use of a vaccine waited until 1954.[4] By the mid-twentieth century, when effective treatments became available, most of the progress had already occurred.[5] In his history of living longer, Steven Johnson says, "Western medicine—for all of its recent achievements—had a miserable track record for most of its existence."[6]

Rather than coming from medical advances, early improvements in health came from rising standards of living, better nutrition, and a strengthening public health movement.[7] A central contribution of public health in the early nineteenth century began with combating the filth and water contamination in cities created by industrialization and urbanization. These efforts promoted healthier lifestyles, an emphasis on prevention, and programs to help the poor and vulnerable. Later public health progress involved ensuring safer food, bringing nursing care to the homes of those in need, understanding the social sources of racial disparities in health, reducing tobacco use, and making vaccines widely available. Today, the emphasis on healthy lifestyles, prevention, and, most obviously, the behavioral changes required by the COVID-19 pandemic is broadly accepted. But the path to this end point was neither swift nor smooth.

The prominence of public health measures in the progress made against disease and death over the past two centuries calls for a story. Advances in public health involved scientific discoveries, vigorous resistance, strong personalities, and new forms of social behavior. And the advances differ from the better-known discoveries of clinical medicine. Public health has traditionally been defined as the science of preventing disease, prolonging life, and promoting health through organized community action.[8] As Virginia Berridge notes, the definition is contested.[9] Its application and activities differ across contexts and time periods, but the emphasis on the community or population rather than individual treatment in a clinic or hospital makes public health distinct. At its core, public health addresses the social conditions under which people live with collective efforts to improve the social, cultural, and physical environments that affect health.[10]

The story begins with two Englishmen in the early nineteenth century, Edwin Chadwick, a lawyer by training, and Thomas Southwood Smith, a minister and physician. They founded what might be called the sanitary movement. The idea they promoted, that health and quality of life could be greatly improved with community cleanliness and hygiene, has become an accepted part of modern life. John Snow refined public health efforts to improve sanitation by showing that cholera was spread through contaminated drinking water. Still later advances came from Harvey Wiley in food safety and Lillian Wald in community nursing. W. E. B. Du Bois stands out for directing attention to racial inequality as a public health problem. Twentieth-century public health brought success in other areas. Richard Doll demonstrated the harm of smoking beyond a reasonable doubt, and D. A. Henderson led global efforts to eradicate smallpox.

The innovators responsible for progress in public health not only saved many from dying and changed the way we live but also led fascinating lives. The discoveries they made and the policies they advocated invariably had opponents. Rather than being welcomed, they had to battle to save lives. Some are famous—most notably Snow and Du Bois—while others are less well known. Yet, all their stories and their accomplishments deserve attention. Each chapter in this book thus presents the life, ideas, actions, failures, and successes of an advocate for public health. Following the lives of these innovators as they ask questions, address puzzles, overcome obstacles, and devise solutions makes their accomplishments tangible, even hundreds of years later.

The history is largely an uplifting one. Despite failures, incomplete progress, and enduring problems of health inequalities, public health advances have improved the lives of countless people. Historians of medicine have moved beyond grand narratives of triumphal and heroic progress against ignorance.[11] What may appear to be discoveries and advances brought about by single individuals most always depended on a network of innovations, actions, and people. These networks included "the work of activists and public intellectuals and legal reformers . . . [and] required new social movements."[12] Nevertheless, the inspirational life stories of these public health advocates whose ideas and actions succeeded in spurring collective efforts to improve the health of populations remain a valuable part of the account.

This book tells these stories, highlighting the theme that advances in public health have made life today considerably healthier, longer, and more satisfying. It interweaves the lives of public health advocates with the context of the times and the progress made against disease. Although based on the scholarly literature (fully documented), the book presents the stories and descriptions of the historical context in a readable, engaging way. It should interest students and general readers as well as public health specialists wanting to know more about the background of their field.

The accomplishments of the past have implications for the present. Many of the problems addressed in the past have reemerged today in altered form. Despite the enormous progress, many places throughout the world, including in rich nations, still suffer from poor sanitation, contaminated drinking water, unsafe food, health disparities, tobacco use, and lack of access to vaccines. Drawing on the lessons of history to guide current policy requires a good deal of care. Simple extrapolations from the past to the present seldom have much value. But one overarching idea links the past to the present. The innovators of the past, much like public health leaders today, recognized the importance of the social determinants of health and the value of organized community action in addressing health problems.

1.

The Obnoxious Bureaucrat
Edwin Chadwick and the Fight against Filth

Edwin Chadwick considered his position in 1848. For the past decade, he had worked ceaselessly to improve the cleanliness of English cities. He fought corrupt local officials, badgered the prime minister and members of Parliament, gathered reams of data on living conditions and sickness across the country, maneuvered around other political appointees in charge of public health, and devoted long days and nights to his goals. He was only a bureaucrat, appointed for fixed terms on committees to look into public health problems. But he made the most of his tenuous position.

In his view, he had done more than anyone else to improve the health of English citizens.[1] He was the strongest advocate of the sanitary idea—that sickness comes from living in squalid, filthy environments. He had led what would later be called the sanitary movement to clean up unhealthy living conditions. He had written the best-selling report describing the sewage and garbage that surrounded the people living in the poorest areas of cities. He had roused public concern when his report had been ignored or over-

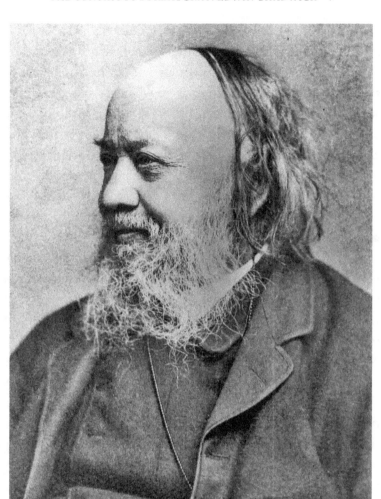

Edwin Chadwick. *Source:* Wikimedia Commons, from the London School of Hygiene and Tropical Medicine.

looked by most of the middle-class and rich citizens in the country. He was the one who had devised engineering schemes to remove waste efficiently and improve access to clean water. He was the one who pushed hardest for the new sanitation law that Parliament had just passed.

Nonetheless, his enemies often frustrated his goals. Not only the corrupt officials and self-interested politicians who had watered down the new law but also members of the medical profession. Chadwick thought doctors were wholly unsuited to understand the problem of public health.[2] They dealt with individual patients, and however much they helped these patients, they could not do much to deal with the larger problem of unclean living conditions. Perhaps worse, the physicians concerned about public health and living conditions got credit that was due to him.[3] It might be too strong to call him "doctor-hating,"[4] but the resentment was deep.

Dr. Thomas Southwood Smith, a minister and physician, had been the first to call for more sanitary living conditions.[5] Chadwick could recall that Smith had introduced him to the problem with a visit to a London slum.[6] Smith recognized the benefits of sanitary conditions early on and did laudable medical work in fever dens and hospitals. As a physician, however, Smith was devoted to patient treatment. In Chadwick's view, he lacked the organizational capacity, leadership skills, and disposition for action. Doctors did not really address the underlying sources of sickness and disease.[7] Chadwick knew that he was the one who implemented the ideas and deserved the major credit. Identifying the problem was easy enough; the real work was to correct the problem.

Despite his good efforts and successes, Chadwick knew that many disliked him. He was once called "the most hated man in England."[8] Charles Dickens, England's most popular writer, snubbed Chadwick but praised Smith.[9] The politicians looked to Smith for guidance and leadership. Chadwick worried about his reputation. Who would get credit for the sanitation innovation? Who would be remembered?

Eventually, Chadwick would be celebrated as the force behind the sanitary movement. He would be knighted by Queen Victoria, and long after his death, historians would write books about his accomplishments. But success did not come easily. The problem of public health in England during the first half of the nineteenth century required radical change—and an obnoxious, arrogant, and persistent bureaucrat to push for the change.

Life in Industrial England

Industrialization in England and elsewhere brought a common set of problems. The wide-scale growth of factories and mass production of goods emerged first in England—and so did the public health problems. The population of Britain grew remarkably during the earlier periods of industrialization, rising from five million to nine million people from 1700 to 1801.[10] Factories concentrated thousands of workers in small areas. The large equipment and steam-powered generators could not be moved to where the people lived, so people came to live near the factories. Many came without jobs and resources, attracted by the vague hope of finding employment. Those that did have jobs received miserly wages and had little job security. In rural areas where parents had many children, the lack of land for the offspring led to migration to cities. Inevitably, the supply of workers outstripped the available jobs and lowered wages. While poverty was always present in rural areas, its concentration in industrial cities was unprecedented. Not only was it more obvious when concentrated in cities but, as Karl Marx and many others recognized, the poverty seemed all the worse in comparison with the growing wealth in nearby affluent areas of the cities.

In terms of health, poverty combined with overcrowding to create squalor in the growing towns and cities. Feces, garbage, and sewage could be easily buried or washed downstream in small rural towns where land was plentiful and people were spread out. The same practices of dumping waste and garbage into the streets, backyards, nearby cesspits, and local streams and bodies of water would not work in cities. The sheer number of residents simply exceeded the capacity to flush out the environment. There were no pipes for water or sewage, little in the way of garbage collection, and few government services. At best, the refuse dumped into the street would occasionally be swept up into a dunghill and sometimes purchased and moved away in carts.[11] More commonly, all kinds of filth surrounded the people who lived there.

Bill Bryson in his characteristically entertaining "short history of private life" illustrates in gruesome detail some of the problems.[12] Most people urinated and defecated outside or used chamber pots for their waste, which they stored in cupboards in bedrooms or dining rooms before dumping the contents into cesspits. Night soil men were hired to clean out the cesspits with buckets—an obviously unpleasant task that those in poor neighborhoods could not afford. The expanding cesspits then tended to overflow into yards, houses, and streets. Worse, cesspits were designed to let water leak out at the bottom, leaving a thicker sludge that was easier to dispose of. Unsurprisingly, the leakage could mix into wells and water supplies. Sometimes cellars of houses would become filled with human waste.

If that wasn't enough, butchers discarded unused animal blood and guts in much the same way, and horse manure filled most streets. Food needed to be protected from the swarms of houseflies attracted by the waste. Even then, people complained that food had "the strong taste of the dunghill left by the flies."[13] With rain, waste would wash into nearby streams and rivers. The main river in London, the Thames, had an overpowering stench that led the famous physicist of the time, Michael Faraday, to call the river "an opaque brown fluid" and "a fermenting sewer."[14] Travelers said they could smell London from miles away.[15] A cartoon from that time—"Death Rows on the Thames"—illustrates the concerns of London residents about the filthy and dangerous water.

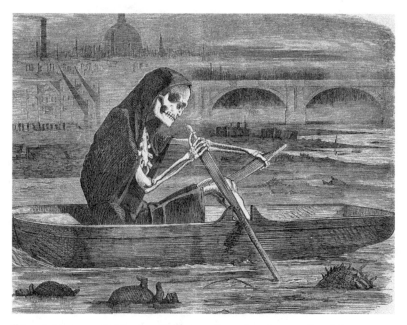

"Death Rows on the Thames." Cartoon from *Punch* magazine, July 10, 1858. *Source*: Wikimedia Commons.

Another problem came from local graveyards, usually situated around the parish church.[16] Local churches received fees for burying the dead on their grounds, and villagers believed that a church burial was holy and respectful. With such strong demand, churchyards became overfilled with dead bodies. New coffins and bodies were stacked on top of old ones, graves tended to be shallow, and corpses could be easily displaced. Heavy rains could wash organic matter into the streets, local wells, and nearby streams and rivers. Even those unaware of germs and disease could understand that mixing decaying bodies with water runoff posed a health risk. Nevertheless, both local parishes and relatives of the deceased resisted any change in traditional burial practices.

Population growth and crowding made cleanliness nearly impossible. Bryson again gives examples. An infamous slum in London contained 54,000 people packed into just a few streets; 1,100 people lived in twenty-seven houses along one alley (40 per dwelling), and one house in another neighborhood had 63 people living together.[17] Privies or outhouses were rare in poor neighborhoods. One area in Manchester had two for 250 people.[18] Those without access to privies just used their backyards.

Although death rates were starting to fall overall during this period, crowded cities were an exception to the trend. The rates rose in growing industrial cities such as Birmingham, Bristol, Liverpool, and Manchester.[19] Regular epidemics of cholera and typhus terrorized city residents. They emerged suddenly and spread quickly. Things had improved since the Great Plague in 1665–1666, and a vaccination for smallpox had been developed, but other disease epidemics continued to kill large numbers of people in the early 1800s.[20]

Doctors at the time recognized that resurgent epidemics came from the increases in crowding and filth among the growing numbers of people stuffed into the poorest districts.[21] But they could do little. They could recommend that sick patients be quarantined, get plenty of rest and liquids, and receive constant care from family members. But such recommendations were seldom practical in poor and crowded parts of the city.

An Obsession with Order

During this time of worsening public health, Edwin Chadwick stumbled across the one great idea of his life—the sanitary idea—by almost dying. While training to be a lawyer, he made friends with a group of young men devoted to a new philosophy of social life, a philosophy based on rationality, order, and human happiness. One member of the group, Dr. Thomas Southwood Smith, took Chadwick on a tour of several fever dens in the London slums—the poorest, dirtiest, and most disease-prone places in the city.[22] Chadwick was no stranger to the underlife of London. As a lawyer in training, he visited prisons and workhouses, had regular contact with criminals, and could walk to nearby rookeries (a slang term for a dense collection of housing typical of slum areas).[23] The disease and poverty he saw were both fascinating and appalling. With his new friend, he would have the chance for an even closer look at the disease-ridden and ravaged lives of the city's indigent residents.

On one visit to the East End of London—the most notorious slum area of the city—he contracted a fever and almost died.[24] Biographers provide little detail about this event, but it must have greatly affected his views. He was healthy, with adequate income and nourishment, and he did nothing to make himself vulnerable to disease. Yet, a visit to places where disease was common nearly led to his death. A simple implication followed: Disease does not come from poverty itself but from the squalor and filthy conditions in which people were forced to live. Fever thrived there and potentially could affect, as epidemics regularly did, everyone living in the city. The filth had to be eradicated.

Chadwick's insight was by no means unique to him. It would have been obvious to almost anyone looking carefully at the conditions. Dumping garbage and human waste into the street, letting water from the street drain into wells and drinking water, and building houses over cesspools of liquid waste and sewage could not be wise. Chadwick had something more than an idea about filth and disease, though. He had a drive for order and efficiency.[25] He wanted a system of sanitation based on logical organization and rational thinking. He appears to have had little love or pity for the people exposed to these conditions, and he lacked a strong sense of charity,[26] but he desperately wanted to clean up English cities and towns.

By all accounts, Chadwick was an easy man to dislike. He was said to be egoistic, despotic, tactless, intolerant, combative, uncompromising, impatient, rude, arrogant, overbearing, insensitive, and impossible to work with.[27] He has been de-scribed as having no sense of humor and known chiefly for un-necessarily making enemies. A person must be special to de-serve such epithets.

Other observers were only slightly less negative; they portrayed Chadwick as a bore.[28] He would talk incessantly about his ideas for improving the sanitation of towns and cities, oblivious to the lack of interest others had in the topic. Or he was prone to lecture those who failed to understand the importance of his ideas. As most of his proposals involved the subject of human waste, his conversation was not welcome in polite society. It was bad man-ners to talk about a topic that most people then and still today pre-fer not to discuss. Chadwick's obsession shows in his description of one vacation:

> My vacation has been absorbed in visiting with Mr. Smith and
> Dr. Playfair the worst parts of some of our worst towns. Dr. Playfair
> has been knocked up by it and has been seriously ill. Mr. Smith has
> had a little dysentery. Sir Henry De la Beche was obliged at Bristol to
> stand at the end of alleys and vomit whilst Dr. Playfair was investi-
> gating overflowing privies. Sir Henry was obliged to give it up.[29]

Chadwick was special in more positive ways as well. Most obviously, his prickly combativeness and domineering personal-ity were put to use for a good purpose. He was remarkably ener-getic and hard working toward his goals. His ten- to twelve-hour workdays wore out his colleagues.[30] While others might care for music, art, and leisure, and think deeply about spirituality and the meaning of life, Chadwick had little interest in such pursuits.[31] His organized mind and inexhaustible energy led to a single-minded devotion to work.

These traits proved particularly well suited to gathering and re-porting data. He could meticulously work through volumes of government figures. He traveled throughout the country to observe the people and their problems and could convincingly summarize the overwhelming detail in his writings. In person, he was tall and well-built and had great physical strength.[32] His commanding appearance along with his domineering personality must have made him a particularly challenging enemy for the many people he offended.

He did have a happy marriage and family life. He married Rachel Dawson Kennedy in 1839, a woman opposite in temperament. As Finer describes her, "She was all that he was not—charming, witty, with a great sense of fun."[33] His two children were both successful.[34] The son, Osbert, became a civil engineer who focused on public works and sanitation not only in England but also in India, Hong Kong, and other English colonies. His daughter, Marion, became a leader in the women's rights movement. After Chadwick's death, Marion wrote a touching tribute that recognized the difficult character of her father but also the warm and human side he showed to his family.[35]

A Radical Philosophy

The model for his career and influence emerged early. While studying law, Chadwick needed extra money to support himself, and journalism provided some short-term earnings.[36] Among the many articles he wrote, one published in 1828 on insurance and one published in 1829 on policing introduced themes he would return to repeatedly.

The piece on life insurance detailed the evidence supporting what seems today to be an obvious thesis, that people would live longer in a cleaner, healthier environment.[37] It called for the government to improve living conditions with new programs and to collect accurate statistics that would guide officials implementing the program. These actions would help in "removing those circumstances which shorten life, and in promoting those under which it is found to attain its greatest and most happy duration."[38]

The article on policing, like the one on insurance, was also filled with statistics, observations, and personal stories. It noted with dismay that law enforcement in the country lacked a state-run professional police force.[39] Chadwick argued that the police needed to be better organized and to rely on rational principles and knowledge rather than on local traditions and special interests. He further claimed that prevention would deter crime better than punishment by "placing difficulties in the way of obtaining the objects of temptation."[40]

As odd as it may seem, these were radical ideas, and Chadwick fit well into the spirit of the times. As one biographer says of the first half of the nineteenth century in England, "Those were glorious days for a Radical."[41] Radicals favored the reform and rational organization of society rather than the continued reliance on tradition and deference to existing authority. Such ideas had been spreading through France and the United States during the previous century. Chadwick's father had been something of a crusading, though ineffective, advocate of radical change.[42] However, the new ideas came to fruition in a practical way in England during the first part of Chadwick's life. In the 1830s, Parliament passed legislation to end slavery, improve the working conditions of children, and extend the right to vote to about one in five adult men.

As a young man, Chadwick fell under the influence of the intellectual godfather of the reform movement in England. Jeremy Bentham founded a school of philosophy and ethics called utilitarianism. Summarized somewhat crudely, its key tenet is "the greatest happiness of the greatest number . . . is the measure of right and wrong."[43] The philosophy gave primacy to individual freedom and guaranteed rights. Well ahead of his time, Bentham called for the end of slavery, equal rights for women, abolition of the death penalty, stopping the physical punishment of children, allowing married couples to divorce, and decriminalizing homosexual acts.

Chadwick idolized Bentham and subscribed wholeheartedly to his ideas.[44] Utilitarianism offered a principle to determine the best social arrangements, and Bentham's proposed legal reforms would replace the frustrating complexities of the law with order and organization. Chadwick's first real job materialized in 1831, when he became Bentham's literary secretary and moved into his home.[45] At the time, Bentham was writing his *Constitutional Code*, a work that sought to reorganize the government on the basis of reason, efficiency, and utilitarianism. Unfortunately, in 1832, Bentham fell sick, and despite Chadwick's efforts to nurse him back to health, the great philosopher died at age eighty-four.

With Bentham's death, Chadwick was left with legal training that he did not care to use. Instead, he had Bentham's legacy—an ethical social philosophy that he fervently believed would improve the lot of humankind. Although the philosophy fit his desire for order in government and society, he needed a way to apply the ideas. His concern about the harm of an unhealthy environment, published in his article on life insurance, continued. Now was the time to put the ideas to use by imposing some order on the disorganized and unhealthy life around him.

By themselves, however, these ideas generated no income. More than anything, he needed a paying job. Opportunity came from some of his contacts who helped him obtain a government position.[46] Having come from an undistinguished background, he was lucky to be hired. But entrance into the government bureaucracy would, at least to a limited extent, offer the opportunity to move up. Chadwick soon proved his value as a civil servant.[47]

Unfortunately, however, his initial steps would lead to hatred and failure before he gained some success.

Mistaken Ideas

As a result of the problems of industrialization in England, the modern movement to improve sanitation originated there as well.[48] And London, the largest city in England, became the center of the sanitary movement. Other European countries, the United States, and cities across the world would soon follow the lead of English sanitarians such as Chadwick. But the early innovations and improvements in public sanitation came from two mistaken ideas.

The first mistake came from the rudimentary understanding of the causes of disease. One might think it would be evident to all that touching the waste and filth or allowing it to mix with food and water would lead to disease. We know now that waste and filth contain bacteria that cause infectious diseases. However, the theories predominating until later in the nineteenth century, when germs were identified as causes, attributed disease to bad air. The miasma theory held that common diseases and epidemics were spread by noxious vapors that came from rotting matter in the ground.[49] The decay was thought to release poisonous particles that spread through the air, infecting victims even without human contact. One could identify the problem by the unpleasant smell.

Given the connection between unpleasant smells and disease, it was easy to assume the smell caused the disease. Echoing the views of most, Edwin Chadwick stated boldly that "all smell is, if it be intense, immediate acute disease."[50] This idea led many to avoid fresh air and baths that exposed the body to fresh air. While the theory is wrong, it did lead experts to focus on cleaning up smelly areas. Places that smelled the worst—cesspits, dirty streets, and poor neighborhoods—most needed cleaning. Exposed graves, also seen as a source of infected air and rotting smells, needed fixing. Almost by accident, the miasma theory targeted some of the key sources of disease.

The second mistake came from minimizing the role of poverty as a cause of disease.[51] If disease came through the air, as indicated by the smell from waste and decay, sanitation could focus on cleaning up the rot. The people who inhabited these malodorous locales needed no special programs other than to live in a cleaner environment. Chadwick gave surprisingly little attention to reducing poverty as a means of improving health. Poverty was the result rather than the cause of poor sanitation. His single-minded focus on sanitation came more from personal and political reasons than scientific ones, however. He had already worked on the problem of poverty as part of a commission to change the Poor Law. But he garnered mostly criticism and animosity from the effort.

Poor laws in England began in the late 1500s, when local parishes received funds to help provide for their elderly, widowed, and orphaned poor residents. For the impoverished able-bodied and unemployed, the parishes created workhouses that offered food and lodging in return for work. The idea was that workhouses could earn a modest profit by using the labor of their residents, those who could not find jobs to support themselves. For those altogether unable to work, the workhouses provided medical care and childcare.

Workhouses did not want to make conditions too comfortable— that would encourage idleness. Even so, the need was great enough that they often became overcrowded. The overlap and lack of coordination among the boards and commissions running local workhouses made problems worse.[52] Poor relief became inordinately expensive in some places. To keep costs down and discourage participation for all but the most destitute, conditions in the workhouses were allowed, again with the aid of corrupt officials who siphoned funds for their own purposes, to become as awful as possible.[53] As the numbers of poor people in towns and cities grew, the system became even more expensive and unworkable.[54]

By 1832, the Poor Law had become so dysfunctional that a Royal Commission investigated the problems and recommended changes. Chadwick began as one of twenty-six assistant commissioners who would do fieldwork for the commission.[55] He received only token pay but soon distinguished himself. In 1833, he received a promotion to became one of the commissioners.[56] Not surprisingly given his energy and ambition, Chadwick contributed substantially to writing the commission's report.

Among its many recommendations, the report called for the end to outdoor relief and reliance on indoor relief and workhouses.[57] Outdoor relief provided money, food, and clothing to those in need who lived outside the workhouse. It was to be replaced by efforts to help the able-bodied find work. Assistance would be given only as indoor relief—within the workhouses where the people could be regulated.[58] The report also called for a central authority that would frame and enforce regulations for workhouses in a way that created uniformity across the fourteen thousand to fifteen thousand parishes in the country.[59] Chadwick wanted more central control of the parishes and the power to overrule local authorities. He wanted more order and rationality.

Based on the commission's report, the 1834 Poor Law Amendment Act passed Parliament. The amendment sought to save money by restricting relief to the destitute living within workhouses. Although admirable in principle, the new law worked poorly in practice and created fierce opposition. It was viewed as brutal. It also set up a Poor Law Commission to supervise local officials. The commission initially had seven members, plus a paid secretary. Chadwick wanted an appointment as a commissioner but was snubbed. He lacked the background and connections for such a leadership role.[60] Instead, he became the commission secretary. As the position came with a steady salary, Chadwick was pleased in some ways, despite the snub.

Chadwick was blamed for many of the problems of the Poor Law, earning the title "the most hated man in England."[61] He believed that poverty could be deterred by making things even worse for the poor. As one historian summarizes, "The pain of the workhouse was to be greater than the pain of poverty and poor relief."[62] Given his certainty in views and desire for orderly processes, Chadwick attempted to administer the law in an orderly but ironfisted way. The historian Anthony Brundage calls him the "Prussian Minister" for his authoritarian tendencies.[63] He offended those living in poverty by ending needed benefits, offended local authorities by trying to limit their power, and offended politicians and his colleagues on the commission with his inflexible and high-handed manner.[64] His desire for bureaucratic order and efficiency overrode any sense of charity for poor people or respect for local institutions. When he asked to meet with Charles Dickens, the famous author and reformer, Dickens put him off, saying, "I do differ from him, to the death, on the crack topic, the new Poor Law."[65]

Origin of the Sanitary Idea

Likely because of the hostility he created in administering the new Poor Law, Chadwick shifted his focus to sanitation as a special area of interest and expertise. Whatever the reason, he became devoted to the cause. Early biographers tend to treat Chadwick as a trailblazer in the area of public health and sanitation, while more recent biographers tend to view Chadwick as a latecomer who adopted the views of others as his own.[66] One other person who played a central role in the sanitary movement was Dr. Thomas Southwood Smith, the friend who first showed Chadwick some of the fever dens of London.

Some consider Smith to be the intellectual father of the modern public health system, even if he was overshadowed by Chadwick.[67] Well before Chadwick had thought much about sanitation, Smith gave lectures in 1813 and 1815 that proposed disease prevention through improved sanitation. In 1824, he wrote an article on "Contagion and Sanitary Laws" that traced disease to preventable problems in sanitation.[68] Recall that it was around this time that Chadwick, who was studying law, made the acquaintance of Smith. In the 1830s, when Chadwick was working on the Poor Law, Smith published "A Treatise on Fever" and "Report on the Physical Causes of Sickness and Mortality."[69]

As a physician, Smith had expertise and standing that Chadwick lacked. He began his career as a minister in Edinburgh, Scotland, where his congregation grew in large part because of the popular lectures and sermons he gave.[70] After his first wife died at a young age, leaving him with two children, Smith sought to combine the ministry with medicine and began medical studies in Edinburgh. He later moved to England to practice both professions, and in 1824 he was appointed physician to the London Fever Hospital.[71] Over the years, he became attracted to utilitarianism and joined with other advocates. He became close enough to the leader Jeremy Bentham that, in accordance with the philosopher's will, he was given the honor of publicly dissecting the body and lecturing on his observations.[72]

Smith's fame began with the publication of regular lectures that he gave in Edinburgh while serving as a minister. The lectures, published as "Illustrations of the Divine Government" in 1817, not only discussed the sanitary idea but also reflected Smith's religious views that public health had a moral justification. He wrote that to realize God's purpose, "What can be improved, must be improved."[73] If disease and misery that came from poverty were preventable, they must be prevented rather than accepted as God's will. He later became known for his good works. Besides his efforts in the London fever hospital to fight disease, Smith sought to help children working in factories.[74] He had many influential friends, including Charles Dickens, who much admired Smith and his work.[75]

Smith had advantages over Chadwick in gaining the respect of colleagues. He was a physician, while Chadwick was a lawyer and bureaucrat. In terms of personality, Smith was compassionate, with a serene and sweet disposition. He was not interested in money or status and was large-hearted, not at all careful in managing his money. A contemporary, Thomas Powell, wrote that he "deliberately sacrifices a large private practice that he may work for the millions instead of the few."[76] When not working, he enjoyed poetry and music, and relaxed with his second wife and children in the quiet of a rural home outside of London. Smith had faith in the goodness of God and confidence in the innate responsibility of people. If conditions were arranged properly, with kindness and through sanitation, the world would be perfected.

Smith lacked the bulldog personality of Chadwick to promote his ideas. The reputation he gained came from hard work, calmness, and commitment, in contrast to Chadwick's prickliness and political infighting. Smith's sense of charity and trust in people differed from Chadwick's hard-hearted view that people needed discipline and order to overcome greed, laziness, drunkenness, and impulsiveness.[77] According to Chadwick, this discipline could be achieved by proper authorities setting up a system of sanitation and enforcing regulations, thereby improving the lives of people living in poverty. This obnoxious single-mindedness had advantages for the sanitary movement, but it was Smith who received respect and admiration.

Chadwick worked closely with Smith over the years but tended to discount the physician's contributions. Indeed, Chadwick saw Smith as a rival for a position on a sanitation commission.[78] When a newspaper called Smith the real founder of the public health movement, Chadwick objected. He said that the sanitary movement came from his own work on the Poor Law and that Smith's reputation came from his own efforts to help his colleague. He wrote to Smith, "I believe that in every instance in which you have been engaged in similar public service, it has been on my recommendation."[79]

Besides personal jealousy, Chadwick objected to what he viewed as Smith's medical bias. To Chadwick, medical approaches to sanitation focused too much on the patient-doctor relationship. Prevention in his view came more from better engineering and organization than from medical treatment. In a letter to his colleague, Chadwick told Smith that he was unsuited for a position on the new sanitation commission: "I think the position is one incompatible with your habits and that you would fail in it."[80] Chadwick further said: "The immediate and pressing need will be for engineering. The medical demand seems to be collateral."[81]

Despite apparent animosity and petty jealousy, Chadwick had a point. He admitted his debt to Smith and other physicians who advocated for prevention.[82] Nonetheless, fighting disease through sanitation would require a new approach. It would require piped water, new systems of drainage, and rules to properly dispose of garbage. Medical knowledge was needed but not primary. Indeed, given the acceptance of the miasma theory of disease, which would not be fully rejected for many decades, medical knowledge was limited. Implementing sanitation procedures was a political and engineering task. It required political maneuvering and stubborn persistence. Chadwick went so far as to write that curative medicine was a sham,[83] as doctors did little to prevent disease. He contrasted the medical approach with his "strong conviction of the superior importance of the study (as a science) of the means of preventing disease."[84]

That is not to say that medicine brought no benefits. During the early 1800s, the number and quality of physicians had increased.[85] Although still ignorant of the underlying causes of infection, they could do good even with rudimentary knowledge. They could advocate cleanliness, proper bedding and sleep, separation of those with fever from others, and use of some simple medications. Their participation on the sanitary commissions was critical. But Chadwick's point was not that medicine was useless but that it could not keep up with new problems emerging from the growth of cities, industrialization, and poverty. Despite improvements in the practice of medicine, "disease was winning the race."[86]

The historian Christopher Hamlin makes the case that the medical field was unprepared to deal with the social causes of ill health that had reached crisis proportions in the 1830s.[87] Health problems came from filth, hunger, overcrowding, and brutal working conditions, but the medical field—with the exception of physicians like Smith—persisted in standard practices. At a time when they needed to become social experts, doctors continued to treat individual patients in private consultation rather than take on issues of public policy. Further, as Hamlin states, medicine was "a poorly united, overcrowded, and squabbling set of professions."[88] The profession lacked the organized power to enter and shape political debates.

The Sanitary Report

Chadwick's efforts to implement and enforce controversial and unpopular aspects of the new Poor Law made him many enemies.

He was accused, correctly in many ways, of being more concerned with regulation and order than with feelings and compassion for poor people. Others recognized the need to compromise, wisely balance competing interests, and show respect for those with differing views. Chadwick, in contrast, was motivated by uncompromising principle and saw opponents as foolish and ignorant enemies.[89] Given his personality, it was no wonder he angered so many. He certainly felt misunderstood, insisting that he should receive credit rather than criticism for his work on the Poor Law. Eventually, the opportunity to restore his reputation arose.

Focusing on sanitation would avoid the criticism he had received. Chadwick could see that cleaning up towns and cities in ways that would reduce disease would help the those living in poverty. It would improve their quality of life, allowing them to enjoy what the middle classes enjoyed in cleaner parts of towns and cities. While the problem of poverty was intractable, the problem of sanitation resulted from "removable causes."[90] It could be fixed.

In 1838, Chadwick began his great push to improve sanitary conditions. In that year, an outbreak of fever in Whitechapel, a notorious slum area of London with a stagnant pond, spurred church authorities to action.[91] They sought the advice of Chadwick, who went to the Poor Law commissioners. He proposed that a committee be set up to investigate the health problems in Whitechapel and the city more widely. Chadwick and Smith along with two other physicians were appointed to the new commission.[92] They were to report on the conditions and develop recommendations for ways to attack the problems.

Chadwick had to do some maneuvering to get the commission established. It would need the support of other Poor Law commissioners, several of whom detested Chadwick and on principle opposed anything he wanted. Others, however, welcomed the new appointment, being glad to rid themselves of their difficult co-worker.[93] Releasing him to other duties would remove the source of friction. With support from Parliament, the prime minister instructed the Poor Law Commission in 1839 to establish an inquiry into the health of the laboring classes in the city and other parts of England and Wales.[94]

Scholars debate Chadwick's motives in the commission.[95] He certainly viewed it as a step toward his long-term goal of improving sanitation and imposing order on cities and towns. Less charitable views attributed his motivation to personal goals. The shift to sanitation would save his career and reputation from the failures of the Poor Law and the difficulties in its management.[96] Removing health "nuisances" would reduce poverty and the need for poor relief.[97] He could focus on disease-producing conditions that, in his view, led to poverty, rather than on better pay for workers, higher quality housing, and income redistribution. Directing his energy and attention to houses, streets, and sewers rather than to people avoided the issues and problems that the Poor Law addressed so inadequately.[98]

Chadwick began work on the new inquiry into the health of the laboring classes in his usual thorough way. He sent letters to local Poor Law assistant commissioners throughout England, Wales, and Scotland, who then circulated them to other local officials.[99] The letters included a set of questions that requested officials to first visit schools, neighborhoods, hospitals, and homes where deaths occurred most often and the young and old alike were "in the lowest sanitary condition."[100] The officials were asked to describe the conditions of the neighborhoods, particularly the sewers, drainage, and street cleaning. A detailed questionnaire for agencies that compiled statistics was also provided. Chadwick himself gathered information from his wide circle of acquaintances. Upward of two thousand commissioners, medical officers, clerks, inspectors, experts, and others were approached for data.[101] In addition, Chadwick traveled personally to make his own observations and read widely on problems of sanitation and health.

Along with the help of his informants and others on the commission, Chadwick authored a report on the findings. But controversy and resistance surfaced even before it was published. One member of the Poor Law Commission, a long-time foe of Chadwick, objected to the criticisms the report made of local water companies, administrators, medical professionals, and sewage commissions.[102] When Chadwick in turn refused to moderate his harsh assessments, the commission members threated to veto the report. A compromise allowed Chadwick to publish the report under his own name rather than that of the Poor Law Commission.[103] Those opposed to the report avoided any negative response to it but, as it turned out, gained little credit for its generally positive reception. The report was tied singularly to Edwin Chadwick, as was the growing sanitary movement that it sparked. As Jon Queijo says in his study of medical advances, "Today, Chadwick's achievements are viewed as the turning point in the history of modern sanitation."[104]

When some readers later suggested that other members of the commission deserved more credit and that Chadwick was not the sole author, he was greatly insulted. One Dr. Gavin stated at a public meeting in 1848 that Smith deserved some of the praise.[105] Chadwick demanded in a letter that Smith disclaim all such recognition. Chadwick wrote that he was "unaware of any public agitation whatsoever upon the subject" until he called on the commission to investigate the consequences of the fever outbreak in Whitechapel.[106] Critics would say that, despite his important role, Chadwick unfairly dismissed the work of Smith and others.

If others deserved credit for recognizing the importance of the sanitation problem and offering bits and pieces of evidence to support their ideas, the sanitary movement still lacked a leader. Someone was needed to organize the efforts and promote the ideas behind public health. Whatever his motives and dependence on the ideas of others, Chadwick supplied the leadership that was missing.[107] The obnoxious bureaucrat took the initiative in spreading the sanitary idea.

Surprising Popularity

The *Report on the Sanitary Condition of the Labouring Population of Great Britain* came out in 1842. The press generously praised it.[108] Even one of Chadwick's worst enemies on the Poor Law Commission, G. C. Lewis, grudgingly complimented the report, saying, "It contains a great deal of good matter, and on the whole, I prefer it to anything else he has written."[109] To the surprise of many, the report became a best seller. More than ten thousand copies were distributed free of charge, and it went through numerous printings to meet demand.[110] Readers may have been less interested in the principles of sanitation than the vivid descriptions of the filth of cities and the horrible conditions under which their poorest residents lived.

Much of the report's success can be attributed to the remarkable detail and overwhelming evidence of sanitation problems. Many others, including Smith, had presented anecdotes illustrating the pressing need to clean up cities, but careful statistical analysis of the problem had been lacking. The detail provided by the report fit well with a statistical social movement that intensified in England in the 1830s.[111] Statistics could, in the view of social reformers, be applied to social conditions to improve the lot of the disadvantaged. Chadwick filled his report with numbers. Never before had such a systematic study of sanitation and health been done. Along with impressive statistics, the stories and descriptions of the lives of the country's most impoverished inhabitants fascinated readers at the time. The vivid details of these people's living conditions must have shocked middle-class readers, who could not look away from the morbid stories. Chadwick knew how to make a convincing case to the public.

The Problem

Chadwick began with an overview of the toll taken by epidemics and contagious diseases. Aiming for both precision and power, he noted that the annual slaughter in England and Wales from these causes of death reached 56,461 in 1838.[112] If one in ten died from fever, then the effects of disease on those sickened and weakened before they recovered were even more widespread. Chadwick summarized the deadly consequences in a memorable comparison: "the annual loss of life from filth and bad ventilation are greater than the loss from death or wounds in any wars in which the country has been engaged in modern times."[113] And the loss of life primarily affected the young, who otherwise would have lived for many years.

Page after page of quotations came from his local informants, each as gruesome as the others. To illustrate, one local official in Tiverton, a town in southwestern England, described one of its poor districts:

> Before reaching the district, I was assailed by a most disagreeable smell; and it was clear to the sense that the air was full of most injurious malaria. The inhabitants, easily distinguishable from the inhabitants of the other parts of the town, had all a sickly, miserable appearance. The open drains in some cases ran immediately before the doors of the houses, and some of the houses were surrounded by wide open drains, full of all the animal and vegetable refuse not only of the houses in that part, but of those in other parts of Tiverton. In many of the houses, persons were confined with fever and different diseases, and all I talked to either were ill or had been so: and the whole community presented a melancholy spectacle of disease and misery.[114]

He went on to describe the housing:

> Many [cottages] are built on the ground without flooring, or against
> a damp hill. Some have neither windows nor doors sufficient to keep
> out the weather, or to let in the rays of the sun, or supply the means
> of ventilation; and in others the roof is so constructed or so worn as
> not to be weather tight. The thatch roof frequently is saturated with
> wet, rotten, and in a state of decay, giving out malaria, as other
> decaying vegetable matter.[115]

Still another medical officer in the largely rural area of Chippen-
ham said:

> During three years' attendance on the poor of this district, I have
> never known the small-pox, scarlatina [scarlet fever], or the typhus
> fever to be absent. The situation is damp, and the buildings un-
> healthy, and the inhabitants themselves inclined to be of dirty
> habits. There is also a great want of drainage.[116]

In Leeds, according to a Mr. Baker, only 68 of 586 streets were
paved by the town.[117] Those without pavement had little or no
drainage, and the sewers that existed easily became blocked.
Ashes and filth were thick enough to raise the level of the unpaved
streets. Stagnant water often spilled under the doorways of the
houses, and then the privies overflowed into the streets. City governments failed to keep them clean of refuse and waste: "Whole
pools of stagnant water, decayed animal and vegetable matter,
and many other nuisances of a like description lying in heaps from
one end of the street to the other."[118] The standard way of removing waste—human labor by scavengers—worked poorly in deprived areas.

The next step in the logic of the argument was to connect the
squalid conditions to disease. One doctor in Derby described how,
among fifty-four similar houses on the same street, half were afflicted by typhus fever and the other half remained comparatively

healthy. The afflicted half lacked drains, and the cesspits over-flowed into a nearby ditch and formed "foul and stinking pools."[119] The houses of the healthy half were protected by a wall that di-rected the ditchwater to a nearby drainage sewer. Efforts to in-stall drainage systems were primitive. In Liverpool, "The only means afforded for carrying off the fluid dirt being a narrow, open, shallow gutter, which sometimes exists, but even this is very generally choked up with stagnant filth."[120]

Chadwick presented other quantitative information to affirm the connection between poverty and disease, including a table with figures from Paris neighborhoods, presented here as a graph (see below). The trend line shows that neighborhood mortality rises steadily with neighborhood poverty.

Some of Chadwick's other data collectors described how deaths fell when drainage systems were put in place. John Marshall Jr. of Ely noted that that one area of his town was "at one period in a desolate state, being frequently inundated by the upland waters,

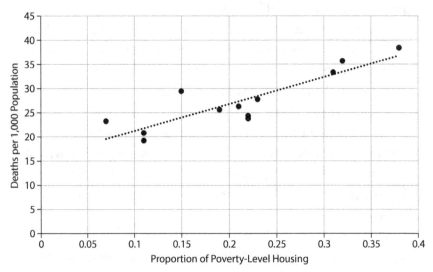

Poverty and mortality in Paris neighborhoods, 1822–1826. *Source:* Data from Chadwick 1842, 171.

and destitute of adequate means of drainage; the lower parts became a wilderness of stagnant pools, the exhalations from which loaded the air with pestiferous vapours and fogs."[121] Now, however, "an alteration has taken place which may appear to be the effect of magic."[122] The use of drainage, embankments, and engines improved the air and stabilized the area. "These very considerable improvements, though carried on at a great expense, have at last turned to a double account, both in reclaiming much ground and improving the rest, and in contributing to the healthiness of the inhabitants."[123] Chadwick also turned to reports from Italy to further demonstrate the benefit of drainage systems. One Italian described the adoption of floodgates in a Tuscan town that "permanently suppressed the marsh, also expelled the fevers."[124]

Given common beliefs that disease spread through the air, Chadwick described the benefits of ventilation. It could help overcome the harm of excess crowding in living quarters and workplaces. He cited one set of dwellings in Glasgow with five hundred people. Although each family had its own room, the lack of ventilation contributed to the constant presence of fever, as many as seven cases a day. After a surgeon fit a small tube into the ceiling of each room to let in pure air, however, "The effect was that, during the ensuing eight years, fever was scarcely known in the place."[125] Similar problems of crowding, poor ventilation, and the fumes from burning candles to give light occurred in dressmaking and hat-making shops, mines, and factories.[126] Windows could be opened but made the rooms too cold in winter. Better ventilation that let in fresh air without exposing workers to freezing drafts improved their health.

The filthy conditions Chadwick described harmed the laboring classes in ways besides poor health. Health problems obviously had economic consequences. Deaths from disease created widows and orphans who became destitute and had to depend on the workhouses and public funds. More costs came from the treatment of patients in fever hospitals, loss of wages from sickness, and medical care in homes. When victims could not pay, government had to pick up the bill.

According to Chadwick, unsanitary conditions further made poor people susceptible to immoral influences. The high risk of death and sickness made them "improvident, reckless, and intemperate, and with habitual avidity for sensual gratifications."[127] These habits in turn meant those exposed to disease cared little about crowding and cleanliness. The crowding together of workers in nearly unbearable conditions lead to depression, and according to one of them, the depression led to excessive use of alcohol: "The natural effect of the depression was, that we had recourse to drink as a stimulant. We went into the shop at six o'clock in the morning; but at seven o'clock, when orders for the breakfast were called for, gin was brought in."[128] Overcrowding of children in unpleasant surroundings led to delinquency among boys, unmarried pregnancy among girls, and poor relationships between wives and husbands. Unlike many others at the time, Chadwick attributed the problems of those living in poverty to the unsanitary environment as much as to flawed personal character.

The Solution

Mr. Byles, medical officer in Whitechapel in London listed the cleanup remedies that he thought were needed. Although they appear commonsensical today, the list nicely summarizes what Chadwick would recommend: "The promotion of cleanly habits amongst the poor; the promotion of sewerage and drainage; having proper supplies of water laid on in the houses; the removal of privies from improper situations. I could point out in our neighbourhood many houses, and some courts, that ought to be pulled down as wholly unfit for human habitation."[129] Chadwick would extend these ideas in presenting his recommendations.

First, neighborhoods and cities needed new drainage systems. The current cleaning system was clearly inadequate. In a conclusion to his review of the evidence, Chadwick began with the obvious: "It is proved that the present mode of retaining refuse in the house in cesspools and privies is injurious to the health and often extremely dangerous. The process of emptying them by hand labour, and removing the contents by cartage, is very offensive, and often the occasion of serious accidents."[130] Moreover, it was expensive and thus unaffordable for poor residents. The wealthy and new-built districts, in contrast, could rely on water closets that discharged refuse through drains into sewers.[131] The use of drains and public sewers in the poorer areas would properly clean the cities and could be done automatically and more cheaply than by human collection. Piping systems ideally would carry the refuse away from streams and rivers, perhaps to farms where waste would be used as fertilizers.[132]

Second, the piping systems needed to be designed so that the flow of waste and sewage would not be blocked. Chadwick's plan was to suspend sewage in water as it was cleared away in piping systems and to replace rectangular brick tunnels that became easily blocked.[133] The report mentioned egg-shaped sewers as a means for smooth drainage, a recommendation he would continue to promote.[134] Engineers who designed and maintained the current system proved vigorous opponents, irritating Chadwick with their unwillingness to see the benefits of his new method.[135] Chadwick argued, "By proper hydraulic arrangements heavy solid substances may be swept away through the iron pipes."[136] The system should also include paving of streets so that rain in wet weather or hoses in dry weather would wash away refuse into sewers and the piping structure. While installing the draining system would be expensive, it would be much cheaper to operate than using human labor.

Third, along with water for flushing sewage, poor neighborhoods needed access to clean water for drinking and cooking.[137] Given the inadequate drainage, most accessible water was impure. There was often no company or organization to provide clean water, or water was owned privately and expensive to purchase. Without nearby access to clean water, families living in many neighborhoods had to walk a considerable distance to fill buckets and jugs, and therefore would sometimes collect water from ditches and reuse dirty water multiple times. Chadwick proposed that a public authority be established to ensure access to quality water at a reasonable price.[138] The authority would build piping systems to carry water into neighborhoods and homes and then reuse the water to convey waste away from where people lived.

Fourth, the system of sanitation should be based on scientific principles and led by experts chosen on the basis of merit rather than political power and patronage. Too often, officials were unskilled and irresponsible—they ignored existing laws that required improvements in cleanliness. In Chadwick's plan, "All new local public works are devised and conducted by responsible officers qualified by the possession of the science and skill of civil engineers."[139] Those with scientific knowledge of the geology of local areas would design drainage systems. A "district medical officer independent of private practice, and with the securities of special qualifications" would be responsible for initiating sanitary measures and executing the law.[140] However, the scientist and engineer would have priority: "Aid must be sought from the science of the civil engineer, not from the physician, who has done his work when he has pointed out the disease that results from the neglect of proper administrative measures, and has alleviated the sufferings of the victims."[141]

Fifth, an orderly and centralized set of laws and regulations was needed. Chadwick's own strong desires for more order plus the rational legal systems advocated by Bentham should be applied to sanitation. Under the current system, local public works were poorly and unequally funded, and spending was inefficient and wasteful. The numerous local districts in charge of sanitation split drainage and water systems that should be integrated. National uniformity was essential for the efficiency Chadwick desired.[142] It provided the only way to overcome the "extensive public loss" following from independent actions and laws of towns.[143] As Chadwick himself was a micro-manager who liked complex organizational schemes, his plans for centrality and uniformity would challenge even the best administrators. On the other hand, the plans would also limit the inequality in sanitation so common at the time.

With these improvements, Chadwick estimated, relying more on guesswork than evidence, that on average a person in the laboring classes would live an additional thirteen years.[144] He further claimed that these classes would improve their morality, becoming more refined in their habits and less tolerant of filth.

Despite the precise numbers, the report lacked high-quality scientific methods. One modern historian reflecting on the report noted that Chadwick misrepresented evidence from the field, suppressed opinions contrary to his own, and, to gain political influence, was intentionally misleading.[145] Unlike scientific approaches, in Chadwick's report "there is the barest pretense of a general induction, much less of a testing of alternate hypotheses."[146] Chadwick was more concerned with promoting sanitation and his career. Recognizing the political nature of the report, he wanted to persuade, and he did so effectively, if not even-handedly.

Partial Progress: The Public Health Act

Even with the popularity of the report, progress toward improving sanitation was slow. Neither the leader of the Conservative nor the Liberal Party wanted the kind of vigorous public health measures that Chadwick envisioned.[147] The usual political battles in Parliament and the government further blocked action. Only after years of debate did Parliament pass the Public Health Act of 1848—a revolution in public health that marked "a commitment to proactive, rather than a reactive, public health.[148] Without the fear of renewed outbreaks of typhus and cholera, supporters and opponents of the law would have debated further. Even so, the act weakened the recommendations of Chadwick's report, particularly in regard to centralization of authority. The act established a General Board of Health but one without funding or power to compel changes.[149] It instead provided loans to local agencies to set up their own boards of health to supervise the building of new drainage and water systems.

It may be that a watered-down version, however much it distressed Chadwick, was necessary at the time. The complex lines of authority across variously defined localities created confusion over responsibilities. Compromise was necessary given the diverse interests involved in sanitation.[150] Chadwick wanted clear organizational authority, but democratic Britain was not yet ready for such a radical change. His goals were too ambitious. But the law did serve to energize some local governments to take responsibility for sanitation.[151]

The new General Board of Health had three commissioners, with Chadwick serving as one of them. Without specified power, the board, and Chadwick in particular, used bullying tactics.[152] The board became increasingly unpopular as a result, and Parliament refused to renew the act after five years.[153] In 1854, Chadwick was forced to retire at age fifty-four (though with a generous pension).[154] The General Board of Health was reestablished on an annual basis until 1858, when its functions shifted to other agencies.

While serving on the commission, Chadwick made one huge mistake. He had recommended piping human waste to farms for use as manure.[155] It proved impractical to build drainage systems out to rural areas, however. The technical requirements were too demanding, and the costs were too high. At the same time, the adoption of newly invented water closets flushed waste and extra water into the sewage system. The plans for safe drainage were quickly overwhelmed. In 1849, a cholera outbreak led Chadwick and others to recommend quick action by "flushing all 'miasmatic deposits' into the Thames."[156] In London, this short-term compromise led to the release of sewage into the Thames, ideally downstream from the center of the city, where it would affect fewer people. Parts of the river nonetheless became "the world's biggest elongated cesspool."[157]

From Chadwick's point of view, this was not a deadly problem. It made the river smell and look dirty but did not directly harm people in the city with dangerous vapors. Done correctly, the sewage would wash away into the vast ocean. Plus, it was a temporary measure that would be corrected when a new system of pipes directed the sewage to rural areas. Little did he know that cholera was spread through infected drinking water and that decades of effort would be needed to clean up the Thames.

The new law was limited in many ways, but it was an impressive first step. He need not have worried about his reputation. Chadwick would receive the credit due for his sanitation efforts. Dozens of books describe his life and works. As Anne Hardy states, "No one could deny Chadwick's role in the founding of modern public health. Whatever else Chadwick was, he was undeniably an active participant in a significant historical process."[158] His misunderstanding of the source of disease and support for flushing waste into large rivers led to disastrous results in the short term. In the long run, however, Chadwick holds a prominent place in the history of public health. Whatever his faults, he identified not only a crucial goal of public health but also the means to reach the goal. The obnoxious bureaucrat, without any medical training, demonstrated the value for public health of government regulations and concerted public action. During his years of service, he did as much as anyone else at the time to improve the health of the public.

Global Sanitation Today

Nearly everyone today shares the goal of the sanitary movement to safely remove sewage from places where people live. Yet many cities in poorer parts of the world face problems similar to those faced by London in Chadwick's time. According to a 2019 report of the World Health Organization (WHO), "Some 829,000 people in low- and middle-income countries die as a result of inadequate water, sanitation, and hygiene each year."[159] Just over half of the world's population, about 54 percent, have access to safely managed sanitation services. About a quarter—two billion people—do not have even basic sanitation facilities such as toilets or latrines. Hundreds of millions end up defecating in the open. The WHO monitors the progress of member nations in improving sanitation and offers risk assessments and program recommendations to deal with the problem. But the growth of urban poor in megacities throughout the world presents a major public health challenge.

Whereas Chadwick and engineers in the mid-1800s struggled to implement sewer systems throughout London, advances in technology promise new ways to deal with global sanitation problems. In 2011, the Bill and Melinda Gates Foundation funded the Reinvent the Toilet Challenge. The goal was to develop and distribute new kinds of toilets that do not require flowing water, a complex system of pipes, and large waste treatment plants.[160] Instead, the toilets seek to convert human waste into burnable fuel and disinfected water on the spot—all without using large amounts of electric power. The challenges of making the toilets affordable and distributing them widely remain, but Bill Gates is optimistic. He expects that the toilet will transform the lives of billions of people across the world. The technology differs, but the goals of the Gates Foundation are an extension of the sanitary movement begun nearly two centuries earlier. As one compiler of medical discoveries acknowledges, "Sanitation is arguably the most important of all medical breakthroughs."[161]

2.

The Disease Detective
John Snow, Cholera, and Infected Drinking Water

Rarely has the reputation of a physician changed so dramatically as that of Dr. John Snow. During his short life of forty-five years—he lived in England from 1813 to 1858—Snow managed to offend the leading physicians and medical experts in London and throughout the rest of the country. He was sometimes ignored, sometimes viewed with condescension, and often vigorously criticized. Medical authorities who held power in the profession said with utter certainty that his writings and the innovative ideas they expressed were wrong-headed.[1] The *Lancet*, "a leading medical journal of the day, considered Snow to be a traitor to empirical medicine."[2] The editor and founder of the journal, Thomas Wakley, was "incensed at what he saw as an attempt to block important public health reforms, [and] accused Snow of unscientific thinking."[3] The short obituary of Snow published in the journal in 1858 barely mentioned his accomplishments and ignored his publications. It said only: "Dr John Snow: This well-known physician died at noon, on the 16th instant, at his house in Sackville Street, from an attack of apoplexy. His researches on chloroform

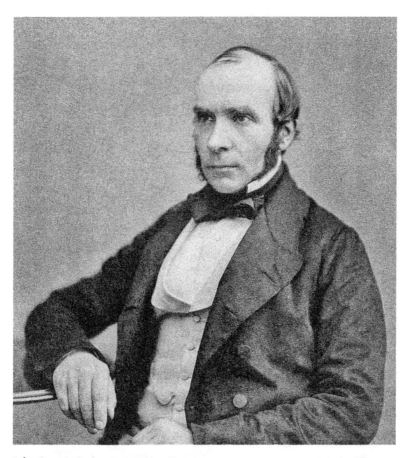

John Snow, 1856. *Source*: Wikimedia Commons.

and other anaesthetics were appreciated by the profession."[4] With only two sentences summarizing his life's work, Snow would appear from the obituary to be either disreputable or unimportant.

What had he done to arouse the antagonism of other medical professionals? He argued that cholera, a disease responsible for killing nearly one hundred thousand people in England during Snow's lifetime,[5] came from drinking water and eating food contaminated by fecal matter. He supported his claims with multiple sources of evidence combined with a single-minded devotion to science. The thought of ingesting fecal matter may have disgusted other physicians, but more important, they felt obliged to defend their own ideas about disease. Once a scientific theory takes hold, the resistance to change is hard to overcome. Snow's claims threatened the widely accepted miasma theory of disease contagion—that disease came from rotting animal and vegetable matter and was spread through the air. Edwin Chadwick, who said that all strong smell is disease, rejected out of hand any ideas that suggested otherwise. Because Snow contradicted the conventional wisdom with his views, most doctors and experts rejected his claims, often vehemently. Worse in the eyes of his critics, Snow was outspoken in opposing policies designed to reduce disease by eliminating stench-producing industries in the city.

Contrast the past views of Snow with those today. He has been called "a genius in epidemiology" with "an elegant, internally and externally consistent theory."[6] In 2003, readers of the medical magazine, *Hospital Doctor*, voted Snow to be "the Greatest Doctor in History."[7] The first professor of epidemiology in the United States called Snow's major publication a masterpiece.[8] The John Snow Society has about four thousand members worldwide, who are devoted to his life and works.[9] The society publicizes his writings, sponsors annual lectures, and sells memorabilia. He is celebrated, considered a medical hero by many.[10] Even the *Lancet* took the opportunity in 2013 to publish an article that corrected the insulting 1858 obituary—155 years later.[11]

Snow took criticism with surprising calmness, simply continuing his work and strengthening the case for his claims. He died well before his ideas were vindicated but likely would have responded to celebrity with the same equanimity he displayed in the face of disapproval. Such a personality was an effective defense against the opposition that new ideas about public health invariably generate. Where Edwin Chadwick responded to critics with hair-trigger anger and bullying, John Snow responded with quiet persistence.

The story of how John Snow and his medical detective work became a model for public health features drama, death, and discovery. The model has not only become a staple of public health and epidemiology but has also made John Snow famous. As a physician, he was experienced in clinical practice. But in trying to understand and prevent epidemics that terrorized England, he became an advocate of public health and a new subfield that came to be known as epidemiology—the statistical study of the incidence and distribution of disease and health.

The Terror of Cholera

The world's largest river delta is found in India and Bangladesh at the mouth of the Ganges River, where it empties into the Bay of Bengal. The delta, consisting of huge tracts of channels, swamps, lakes, and floodplains, is fertile ground. More than 100 million people live in the area, farming the soil and fishing in the waters. It is also a fertile ground for bacteria. The warm temperatures of the area, the ritual bathing of Hindus upriver, the presence of human and animal waste, and the diverse plant and animal life in the delta combine to create ideal breeding conditions for diverse bacterial species.[12] Throughout history, the Ganges delta has been seen as gorgeous, wild, and deadly.[13]

The delta is also the place where the cholera bacteria are likely to have first emerged. The origins are not certain, but early reports of a cholera-like disease in India date back to ancient times.[14] Later, a Portuguese writer described the outbreak of a similar disease in the Ganges delta in 1543. It is not certain if these outbreaks stemmed from the same disease we know today. Christopher Hamlin argues that cholera varied so much across time and place that it is hard to identify a single origin.[15] Even so, most say that a modern form of cholera emerged from the Ganges delta in 1817. It spread through most of India and nearby countries, and then to Europe along common trade routes. It did relatively little damage in Europe, perhaps because of a severe winter in 1823-1824.[16] The spread of the disease during these years is referred to as the first cholera pandemic.

Multiple pandemics followed in the nineteenth century, making their way to Europe and the Americas, often after originating in India and the delta. In England, epidemics occurred in 1831-1832, 1848-1849, 1853-1854, and 1866.[17] The last was the least severe. By the twentieth century, the disease had disappeared from wealthy countries and was limited to more isolated outbreaks in countries suffering from civil wars and natural disasters.

Cholera has been called "the single worst epidemic disease of the nineteenth century,"[18] but in some ways it seems less serious than other plagues. Scholars estimate that cholera caused millions of deaths across the world, while other infectious diseases killed hundreds of millions.[19] At its worst, it was responsible for only 5 percent of the deaths in England and Wales.[20] London was one of the worst affected cities, yet cholera was present for less than two years in total. Other diseases such as typhus, pneumonia, and smallpox killed more people.

More than because of the sheer number of victims, the terror of cholera came from the sudden deadliness of the disease. One vivid description says, "Cholera is a horrific illness. The onset of the disease is typically quick and spectacular; you can be healthy one moment and dead within hours. The disease, left untreated, has a fatality rate that can reach fifty per cent."[21] People could see that cholera killed often and killed quickly—frequently within twelve hours. Not knowing how to prevent or survive the disease, city residents dreaded cholera.[22]

The most obvious symptoms of cholera are severe vomiting and diarrhea. While nasty, the symptoms lead to worse, less easily observed problems. So much water is lost from the vomiting and diarrhea and such severe cramps occur that the heart can no longer pump properly, the blood lacks oxygen to deliver to the body, and the organs can no longer function. Without enough water, the blood becomes thick and capillaries rupture.[23] Cholera was called the blue disease because dehydration and low blood oxygen turned the skin blue.[24] Until the last moments before death, the victim is conscious.[25] One historian notes that no other disease of the nineteenth century had the emotional impact of cholera.[26]

We now know much about the microbiology of cholera. An Italian scientist, Filippo Pacini, first isolated the bacterium in 1854. The Nobel Prize–winning German physician and microbiologist Robert Koch described it in more detail and identified the means of its transmission in 1884. It turns out that cholera is relatively easy to treat. The underlying problem of dehydration can generally be addressed by rapidly administering intravenous fluids and electrolytes or, in milder cases, other forms of oral rehydration therapy. Antibiotics can sometimes speed the recovery and ease the suffering.[27]

Those dealing with the disease in the 1800s, however, knew little. At the time, the reasons why cholera spread so quickly were unknown. Many suspected that a tiny organism caused the disease but relied on guesswork. They did not know how to kill the organism or counter the dehydration it caused. As a result, the fight against the disease had to come from community action and prevention rather than from clinical medicine. Although a physician by training, Snow followed the data in a way that led to a discovery that helped define the emerging field of public health.

An Outbreak in London

Most visitors to London these days make it a point to wander through Soho, one of the city's liveliest neighborhoods, defined by its narrow streets with old buildings and a bohemian feel. The neighborhood contrasts with the beautiful and elegant but uniform white stucco terraces that dominate many parts of London. The buildings in Soho housed clubs in the 1960s and 1970s where, among many others, the Rolling Stones, David Bowie, and U2 played. Still the location of top indie and jazz venues for live music, Soho remains a popular part of the London music scene. Across the street from the tree-lined Soho Square, Sir Paul McCartney located the headquarters of the company he founded to handle his business interests.

Along with places for live music, there are enough bars, restaurants, theaters, and interesting characters to entertain most anyone. Once infamous as the center of the sex industry, Soho now has a less grimy and higher-end appeal. People come from throughout the city to enjoy boutiques and shops, musicals and films, used record stores, food of all types and prices, all-night coffee houses, and gay bars and clubs.

The popularity of the neighborhood makes it an expensive place to live. It continues to have a mix of poor and rich residents but increasingly tips toward the affluent. Most residents of the area likely live long and prosperous lives. The prosperity hides an unpleasant history, however. Centuries ago, poor migrants to London crowded into the area. In fact, in the mid-1800s, Soho became known as a particularly dangerous place to live. It was a center of one of the cholera epidemics that periodically afflicted the city. It also became the place where John Snow gathered evidence to support his theories about the source of these scourges.

Soho has in fact passed through several cycles of gentrification and decline. Steven Johnson describes how Soho was originally built as a part of London where victims of the Great Plague of 1665 could be isolated and then buried. "By some estimates, over four thousand plague-infected bodies were buried there in a matter of months."[28] Cycles of boom and bust followed. During a period around 1700, aristocrats built large homes for themselves in Soho but then deserted the area decades later for newer neighborhoods. Poorer families moved in, with the large homes transitioning into cheap boardinghouses. By the mid-1800s, parts of Soho had become London's most densely populated subdistrict.[29] One of the poor residents, Karl Marx, lived there with his wife, four children, and a maid in a two-room attic. Marx left the cramped quarters during most days to do research and writing at the British Library for his monumental work, *Capital*. But the unpleasant living conditions at home were typical for Soho's inhabitants.

As a poor and crowded neighborhood, Soho was ripe for an epidemic. The area had its share of cesspools to store human waste, and the residents were too poor to pay night soil men to clear them out. Chadwick and other sanitarians gave no special attention to Soho—many other neighborhoods had the same problems. But Soho differed from other London neighborhoods and English cities. It became famous as the center of one sudden and devasting cholera outbreak. That John Snow happened to live and work in the district added to its historical importance.

The Soho outbreak in 1854 began with vomiting and diarrhea in a new baby.[30] Thomas Lewis and his wife, Sarah, lived in a house that was designed for one family but now contained twenty people. Sarah gave birth to a baby girl who at about five months of age began vomiting early one morning. Her diapers contained watery green stools. "Mrs. Lewis had soaked the diarrhea-soiled diapers in pails of water. Thereafter, she emptied the pails in the cesspool opening in front of her house."[31] The cesspool leaked and was only three feet from a well and water pump. The disease passed from the baby's stool to the cesspool and then to the Soho water supply and ultimately to hundreds of others in the neighborhood.

The deadly cholera epidemic in Soho would spread quickly. According to a newspaper article at the time,

> The shopkeepers have dismal stories to tell—how they would hear in the evening that one of their neighbors whom they had been talking with in the morning had expired after a few hours of agony and torture. It has even been asserted that the number of corpses was so great that they were removed wholesale in dead-carts for want of sufficient hearses to convey them; but let us hope this is incorrect.[32]

Even if the stories were exaggerated, some statistics reveal the tragedy of the outbreak: 127 people died in only three days, and 500 people died in about two weeks. As shown in the graph below, the epidemic came on quickly. Snow called it "the most terrible outbreak of cholera which ever occurred in the kingdom."[33]

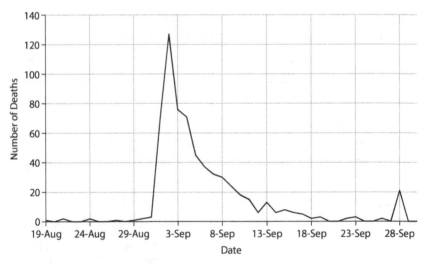

Number of cholera deaths in Soho, London, August 19–September 30, 1854.
Source: Data from J. Snow 1855, 49.

Upwardly Mobile

Given his background, John Snow might never have become a physician. He certainly came from humble circumstances.[34] The first of nine children, he was born in York, England. At the time of his birth in 1813, his parents lived in a poor area of town that was prone to flooding from the nearby river. He enjoyed the good fortune of having an ambitious, upwardly mobile father and mother. His father worked as a laborer and drove a horse-drawn vehicle but must have saved carefully. In 1825, he bought a house in a better neighborhood and eventually purchased farmland. Ownership of land was considered a step up in status.

As Richard Ellis describes it, "Snow's parents seem to have been determined to give their offspring whatever opportunities they could afford in order to better themselves."[35] They allowed their children to attend school rather than requiring them to start working to earn money for the family. With some basic education, the children could take advantage of an expanding economy that allowed those from the lower class to move to the middle class.[36] Many of Snow's younger brothers and sisters also became professionals, finding careers as a vicar, teacher, hotel keeper, and secretary.[37]

As the oldest, John Snow may have enjoyed the most support and opportunity. Certainly, his eventual fame set him apart from his siblings. As one historian says, his rise "from total obscurity to professional eminence and historical renown" was remarkable.[38] At the time, medicine was seen as a way for lower class youth to move up. Becoming a physician required money for apprenticeships and schooling, but the cost was relatively low.[39] It demanded hard work and academic skills to learn anatomy, chemistry, and medicine, but Snow enjoyed hard work, and his skill in mathematics demonstrated his intelligence.[40]

Training to become a physician at the time began with an apprenticeship. The apprentice paid a physician for the chance to learn. Much of the training involved menial work—mixing medicines, taking messages, and making appointments. More usefully, the apprentice also had the chance to see poorer patients and deal with accidents, colds, and fevers.[41] Snow began as an apprentice in 1827, at the young age of fourteen. He spent five years learning from surgeon-apothecary William Hardcastle in Newcastle upon Tyne. He was also among the first students at the new Newcastle School of Medicine in the 1830s.[42] Perhaps Snow's parents or a well-off uncle who lived in Newcastle paid for the apprenticeship.[43]

One experience while Snow was serving as an apprentice stands out. A cholera epidemic came to Newcastle and surrounding areas in 1831–1832. Snow was sent to help victims of the disease in Killingworth Colliery, a small town outside Newcastle.[44] He saw the worst of the disease there—how the diarrhea and vomiting brought suffering and death and how the victims lived in crowded conditions and often worked in mines. His observations would prove valuable many years later.

Snow's personality traits began to emerge during the apprenticeship years. He was intense and reserved with an independent streak that showed in the adoption of practices that were unusual at the time. At age seventeen, he became a vegetarian. He followed the diet religiously for most of his life.[45] The version Snow adopted included drinking distilled water, which was seen as crucial to a healthy colon. The habit was unusual, but Snow was devoted to obtaining pure water. He thought that tap water contained materials that had passed through the human gut and had tiny bits of partially digested meat.[46] No doubt his belief would direct his attention to the quality of public water supplies as a source of disease.[47]

Along with meat, he also chose to abstain from alcohol, another habit he would follow for most of his life.[48] He was quite open about recommending vegetarianism and abstinence to others, even joining a temperance group. Only when suffering from health problems did he, on the advice of doctors, add some wine and animal products to his diet.

He lived and dressed simply. He limited the enjoyment of normal pleasures, instead concentrating his daily life on scientific pursuits.[49] As his friend and biographer, Benjamin Ward Richardson, described it, he "kept no company, and found every amusement in his science books, his experiments, and simple exercise. . . . All who knew him said he was a quiet man, very reserved and peculiar—a clever man, but not easy to be understood."[50] Being so reserved meant he was not eloquent, but he tried to speak clearly and to the point in his lectures and contact with patients.[51]

He was certainly hard-working and industrious.[52] Following a careful schedule, he rose early, worked all day, and retired to bed early. While working, he kept a meticulous diary of his activities and careful records of his experiments and medical cases. He never read novels—from his point of view a waste of time, given his pursuit of scientific goals. He expressed regret about having never married, and he enjoyed the company of children. Even so, a family did not fit his life of discipline, ambition, and hard work.

Medical Education

At the time of Snow's education, the medical profession consisted primarily of physicians, surgeons, and apothecaries.[53] Physicians, the only ones called doctors, had the highest status. Surgeons and apothecaries were seen as a step below doctors. Surgeons were viewed as manual workers and apothecaries as shopkeepers selling medicines.[54] Because Snow first apprenticed to a surgeon and apothecary, he could have practiced after his training as a surgeon and apothecary in a small town. He would not have had to attend medical school.[55]

But Snow, being scholarly and intense, wanted more. After his apprenticeship, he worked as a doctor's assistant for thirty months, this time with pay. Living simply as he did, he saved money for further medical education.[56] In 1836, he began medical school in London while also starting to practice in local hospitals. The rudimentary practice helped provide money during his time of medical study. He rented a house on Frith Street in Soho, where he could see patients. Eight years later, in 1844, he passed the MD exam and officially became a doctor.[57]

It was a long process, considering that he started as an apprentice in 1827, but Snow had reached the top of the medical profession—a long way from his humble beginnings. Because he did not attend Oxford or Cambridge, he still was considered something of an outsider.[58] But he played a prominent role in the Medical Society of London and belonged to many other medical groups.

From the start of his medical career in London, Snow stood out from the norm. First, he published scientific papers based on his observations of patients and treatments. For example, two of his articles appeared in the *Lancet*—one on arsenic as a preservative of dead bodies in 1838, and another on mechanisms of respiration in 1839.[59] It was unusual for practicing physicians to publish any papers and even more impressive to publish papers on the diversity of topics that Snow did.[60] Second, he liked tinkering with medical equipment. Early in his career, he helped develop an inhaler to assist newborn babies in breathing.[61] His attention to improving equipment fit well with a new generation of physicians who were not content to follow the long-accepted wisdom of earlier generations. They wanted to use science and technology to improve medical care.[62] Third, he developed a specialization in the new field of anesthesiology. Given that patients could afford to pay little to doctors, a specialization in anesthesia provided a skill in high demand. It helped establish his practice and pay his bills.[63]

His innovative and skillful work with anesthesia led to some prominence. He became what many viewed as the world's first professional anesthetist.[64] On hearing about the use of inhaled gases to eliminate pain during surgical treatment, Snow learned all he could about the properties of the gases and the equipment to deliver them.[65] He soon became an expert on chloroform, devised improvements in inhaling equipment, and skillfully delivered anesthesia. As a sign of his success, he was twice called to deliver chloroform to Queen Victoria, once for the birth of Prince Leopold and once for the birth of Princess Beatrice. The queen "expressed herself as greatly relieved by the administration."[66] Other physicians recognized his accomplishments in this area, as Snow published several important papers on the topic.[67]

According to Richardson, he administered anesthesia some 450 times annually over the ten years preceding his death. Although anesthesia was a major source of his income, Snow never made much money—only £1,000 a year at most. He often provided services for free.[68] But the work was enough to support his modest lifestyle and give him time for other research. An unintended benefit was that the experience with gases made him skeptical of the miasma theory of disease contagion, which posited the harm of inhaling unpleasant smelling air.[69]

None of these accomplishments compare with what we view today as his major insight on the source of cholera epidemics. It is ironic that what made Snow most famous and successful during his lifetime would be considered a sidelight today, while what offended many and was rejected by most while he was alive ended up making him one of history's greatest physicians.

Statistics and Shoe Leather

Three major cholera epidemics in Britain, 1831–1832, 1848–1849 and 1853–1854, overlapped with Snow's medical career. The first epidemic gave him a hint about the causes of cholera. The second, which killed more than fifty-three thousand in England and Wales, greatly concerned the medical community. The deaths from this epidemic helped Snow develop a clear explanation. The third outbreak, which killed about twenty-three thousand in the country, provided strong evidence for his explanation.

Initially, much of his insight came from simple observations and clear thinking. He was able to obtain some reliable data by 1849 and published his views in a pamphlet titled *On the Mode of Communication of Cholera*. This short document of only thirty-one pages is filled with examples and clear reasoning in support of his views. But with only a few tables and numbers to support the examples, it lacked the detail needed to convince many. The initial evidence appeared incomplete.[70]

More systematic work came in 1855, soon after the third British epidemic, when Snow published a second edition of *On the Mode of Communication of Cholera*. This edition combined the original pamphlet with new material from papers he had published and new data he had found. As Richard Freeman describes it, the volume mixes statistics and shoe leather, mathematics, and detective work.[71] It involved the analysis of data in the privacy of his home and the extraordinarily hard work of getting out into the street to talk to people, ask questions, and see for himself how the disease came to affect local neighborhoods. His analyses provided a model of how to test hypotheses on public health topics.

The evidence he found falls into three rough categories. He used commonsense observations and logical reasoning; he created an insightful map visualizing the source of one cholera outbreak; and he compared the disease prevalence across homes receiving different sources of water. The multiple types of evidence, from different sources and using different data, made a powerful case that cholera was spread in two ways—from personal contact and contaminated drinking water.

Commonsense Observations and Logical Reasoning

Although Snow was busy with his medical practice and research on anesthesia, the 1848–1849 epidemic attracted his attention. The sudden deaths of tens of thousands of people from a frightening disease was obviously concerning. More than that, however, he might have thought that he could make a special contribution. For one thing, his experiments with chloroform and breathing likely led him to question the belief that disease was spread by gaseous vapors.[72] For another, his belief in the value of pure drinking water likely led him to suspect the role of contaminated water.

Whatever the source, Snow's initial hunches made good sense. His reasoning seems so obvious that one would expect others to have drawn the same conclusions. Consider an early example. In his initial visits as a seventeen-year-old apprentice to a town stricken by cholera in the winter of 1831–1832, he could not help but notice that the epidemic hit coal miners hard.[73] Snow watched as miners were brought from the mines after an attack of the disease during their workday. What stood out in hindsight was that, unlike other workers above ground, the miners had no toilets or running water to use when working. They not only defecated in the mines, but they also ate their meals in the mines without washing their hands.[74] The link between human waste, food, and cholera offered only a hint, but it must have been enough for Snow to think differently about the disease. It certainly did not seem that putrid air blowing from distant places would explain the spread of cholera among miners.

Perhaps based on his research on respiration and anesthesia, Snow had another insight. He knew, as did everyone acquainted with the vomiting and diarrhea of the disease, that the poison disturbed the stomach and intestines. If the disease affected the digestive system, it likely must enter the body through the mouth and travel into the stomach and intestines. That seemed obvious. This reasoning, however, contradicted the miasma theory of disease. If disease spread through the air, it would enter the body through breathing and travel into the lungs and blood. Doctors were looking for the cause of the disease in the wrong part of the body.

Snow pointed out a fundamental error in the logic of cause and effect made by some experts. Doctors knew that the blood of cholera victims became thickened. That made it harder to breath and get oxygen to the body. The failure of the organs from lack of oxygen ultimately killed the victims. But Snow pointed out that the changes in the blood followed rather than preceded the vomiting and diarrhea.[75] The loss of water—the vomit and stools were mostly water—caused rather than resulted from changes in the blood. Dehydration of victims came after the entrance of the disease through the mouth and into the stomach and intestines. Thickened blood, trouble breathing, and organ failure then followed.

Neither Snow nor anyone else knew of germs and their role in disease. But Snow had an intuition consistent with germ theory. He believed that the source of cholera, whatever it was, could be swallowed. It would then attach itself to the membrane of the small intestines and multiply.[76] The body attempted to expel the disease with vomiting and diarrhea. Others coming in contact with the sick person could inadvertently be contaminated by the disease. Minute quantities could soil the hands, get into food and drink, and be swallowed.

Snow made other observations consistent with this view of how the disease spreads. Rather than being carried on the air from distant locations, the disease appeared to spread via human contact or, Snow's words, "human intercourse." It came to a new location with travelers from somewhere else where the disease was prevalent. It traveled neither faster nor slower than people traveled and always appeared first at a seaport.

Indeed, the first documented case of the 1848 epidemic occurred at a seaport.[77] A seaman named John Harnold came to England from Hamburg, Germany, a city with an ongoing cholera epidemic. He let a room in a lodge, where he shortly died of the disease. Then eight days later, a man named Blenkinsopp came to the same lodge and slept in the same room. He also died of cholera. Snow says, "Who can doubt that the case of John Harnold, the seaman from Hamburg, mentioned above, was the true cause of the malady in Blenkinsopp."[78] Making the case even more strongly, Snow cites example after example of how the disease spread from a sick person to a healthy one. Even when cholera appeared to emerge anew, without any contact with others who were sick, persistent detective work could find a sick person who was the source.

The claim that the disease passed from sick person to healthy person explained the quick spread of the disease in poor neighborhoods. The crowded conditions made for more contact between the sick and healthy. Of course, the affluent could get the disease as well. But their spacious homes, cleaner neighborhoods, and healthier food and water afforded them more protection than poor people enjoyed. The same logic about personal hygiene could also explain the fact that doctors rarely caught cholera from their patients. They visited patients but did not live with them in crowded conditions and took care to wash their hands after contact with cholera sufferers.

That cholera was spread through personal contact was only one part of the story. Contact could explain the transmission from sick persons to family members, neighbors, and co-workers. But how could it advance quickly over vast areas, in places where contact was limited? Snow had an explanation: cholera was spread through drinking water containing the disease. Dirty water contaminated by victims would be disposed of outside the home, permeate the ground, run along channels and sewers, and get into wells and rivers. This means of contagion, although disputed by many, proved crucial for understanding the disease.

Mapping and the Broad Street Pump

Today, a non-working water pump sits on a busy street in Soho next to the John Snow pub. As Snow was a teetotaler for most of his life, having a pub named after him is one of history's ironies. But the nearby pump serves as a landmark in medical history. The Broad Street pump is famous enough to be listed in guidebooks and on the Trip Advisor website as one of the thousands of sites to see in London (although Broad Street is now Broadwick Street). Its fame comes from John Snow's investigation into the source of cholera in Soho, and his finding that most of the cases there came from drinking well water drawn up by this pump.

The Broad Street pump was located near the center of the area in Soho where in 1854 the sudden and terrifying cholera epidemic occurred. Snow noticed that, of the eighty-three deaths over three days of the outbreak, nearly all occurred a short distance from the pump.[79] Other deaths occurred farther away, but on investigation, it turned out that family members had used the pump. Some had children who attended school near the pump and drank its water.

Despite the reliance of the neighborhood on the well, Snow managed to convince municipal officials to remove the pump handle so residents could no longer draw from the well and risk infection from the water. Officials did not decide to disable the pump impulsively. The well was convenient for a large number of Soho residents. Most did not want to walk longer distances to other wells and carry water back home. Besides, Snow admitted that, although the pump water had an offensive smell, one could see impurities only on very close inspection.[80] When Snow told the officials that the water was contaminated with cholera, they were incredulous but nonetheless had the good sense to take the precaution of having the pump handle removed.

Later, Snow created a simple map of the Soho outbreak that made his case more strongly. The map has since become one of the most famous in public health history. At the time, mapping was seen as a new scientific tool for understanding disease epidemics. As part of the new generation of physicians devoted to innovation, Snow saw the benefits of this tool.[81] He believed that a map could make the patterns of deaths more real than a list of statistics. He proceeded to plot the location of cholera deaths in the Soho neighborhood over a six-week period (August 19 to September 30, 1854).[82] Small black rectangles on the map showed the locations of fatal attacks, and a black circle near the intersection of Broad Street and Cambridge Street indicated the spot of the Broad Street pump. Snow also noted the location of other nearby water pumps.

The map showed the clustering of black marks around the pump. The largest number of deaths occurred on the same block and same street as the pump. Streets with easy access to the pump had many marks, while branching streets that made it harder to get to the pump had fewer. The other pumps showed few nearby deaths. Only one, the Broad Street pump, stood out.

The map also identified exceptions, such as buildings near the pump where few cholera deaths occurred.[83] The exceptions turned out to strengthen the evidence. A workhouse near the pump was surrounded by houses with cholera deaths, but of the 535 workhouse inmates, only five died from cholera. Snow discovered that the workhouse had its own water supply and never sent for water from the Broad Street pump. A nearby brewery had no deaths

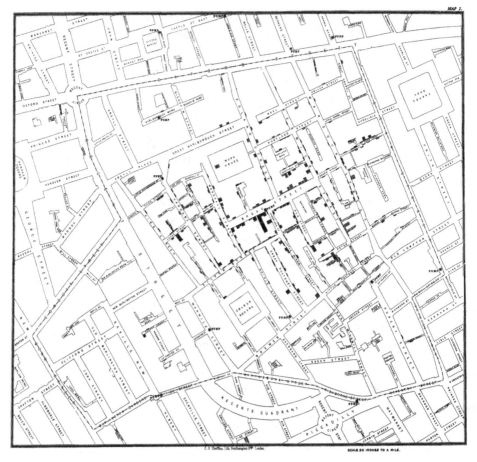

John Snow's map of 1854 cholera deaths in Soho, London. *Source*: Wikimedia Commons, from the UCLA Department of Epidemiology.

among its workers. Taking advantage of their jobs, the workers drank malt liquor rather than water from the pump. In contrast, workers at a nearby factory drank water from a tub filled by the pump. Eighteen of the two hundred workers died from cholera.

Many others lived and died elsewhere, but with enough detective work, Snow could trace their cholera deaths to the pump. For example, a gentleman from Brighton came to Soho after his brother's death. He briefly visited his brother's home, enjoying a small tumbler of brandy with water from the pump. He soon left Soho but died the next evening in another part of London.[84] A widow living in Hampstead, several miles away from the pump, died of cholera. The town had clean water, but it turned out that, having lived with her husband in Soho years ago, she had water delivered to her from the Broad Street pump.[85] A Mr. Gould, an eminent ornithologist living in Soho, normally drank from the pump but was out of town when the outbreak began. On returning and sending his assistant for water, he was surprised to find it had an offensive smell. While Gould declined to drink the water, a servant drank a good deal of it and got sick from cholera.[86]

Many found one additional piece of evidence to be convincing. After the removal of the handle, which ended the use of the water from the well, the number of new cases diminished. The change was not sudden, as those who had drunk the contaminated water earlier died after the handle was taken away. But a chronology revealed a steady decline of deaths on the days after people stopped drinking the water.[87] Snow admitted to limitations of the evidence—so many people had moved from the area that the outbreak may have slowed anyway. If not conclusive proof, the trends before and after the removal certainly fit Snow's claims.

Snow concluded that no other explanation besides the contamination of the Broad Street well-water could account for the pattern of the deaths shown by the map. The suddenness and high death rate of the outbreak suggested a dense contamination of the water. The adjacent leaky sewer was the likely source. In hindsight, the map was crucial for persuading others about the source of the Soho cholera outbreak and the disease more generally. Experts point out that the map, by itself, did little to prove the validity of Snow's thesis. But visualizing the problem made it easy to understand and legitimized the value of other evidence.[88]

Natural Experiments

Combined with the map, the Soho evidence was powerful but still not fully convincing. Snow identified an association between living near the smelly water of the Broad Street pump and dying from cholera during the 1854 outbreak. He also explained the exceptions, such as the lack of disease in a brewery, a workhouse, and streets that did not use water from the Broad Street pump. However, critics would claim that the disease was spread through the air around the pump. Isolation in a brewery or workhouse simply kept workers and residents from being exposed to the air. Snow needed to show something more—that among homes afflicted and unafflicted by cholera, the only major difference was the water they used. If home dwellers all breathed the same air but differed in their drinking water, then the water rather than air must be the cause of the disease.

The third type of evidence provided this information. It took the form of a natural experiment in which some homes received high-quality water while nearby neighbors did not. Experiments today evaluate the effectiveness of new drugs and medical procedures, but these trials have the advantage of being able to randomly assign subjects to a treatment group receiving the new drug or procedure and a control group receiving the placebo or usual procedure. Snow could not ethically assign subjects to drink contaminated water, but he found that in an analogous way residents of London had been assigned naturally to treatment and control groups. Although not a true randomized trial, the natural experiments Snow reported constituted strong evidence.

Take a simple example from 1849 that illustrated the strategy. Two groups of nearby houses in Horsleydown, London, seemed alike, as they were located on either side of a court or alley. Yet, one side experienced "fearful devastation" from cholera, while the other side had only one death.[89] There appeared to be one major difference. On the side of the court with many cholera deaths, residents would wash the linens of cholera victims, then dump the dirty water into a channel where it mixed with well water. The well for the other side of the court with few cholera deaths was better protected and remained relatively clean. All the houses might have noticed a disagreeable odor, but only one side was severely affected by cholera.

These and several other similar examples led Snow to search for more systematic data. As early as 1832, cholera deaths appeared to be related to neighborhood use of river water.[90] In parts of London directly south of the Thames River, cholera death rates were higher than in other parts of the city. This fact was known, but only Snow focused on the varied water sources of the neighborhoods. The Thames River flows through the middle of London and provides water for large parts of the city. However, the water supply for South London came from a part of the river directly below a site for disposal of sewage. Other parts of London got their water from farther upriver, above the sewage discharge.

The attention to drinking water from the Thames River followed from Snow's observations that diseased water entered the body through swallowing. The mixing of sewage into the Thames supported Snow's claim that the cholera disease agent contaminated drinking water. The logic explained the spread of the disease and the high rates of infection in South London. Because the waste and disease in river water was less concentrated than it might be in well water, cholera spread less suddenly and violently than in Soho, and it was dispersed over a wider area.[91]

Snow began with a table displaying the mortality from cholera and the source of the water supply in thirty-eight neighborhoods in 1849.[92] Private companies supplied water at the time. Every district relying on companies that drew water from near the sewage discharge had higher cholera fatality rates than districts relying on water from companies that drew water from cleaner parts of the river. For example, the source of water for fashionable parts of London came from the Chelsea Water company, which took great pains to filter the water. In contrast, the water companies for the disease-stricken poorer neighborhoods south of the river supplied the water "in a most impure condition."[93] The geographic comparison of neighborhoods represented an early form of what today is called the ecological analysis of disease.

Fortuitous changes made in 1852 allowed for a more rigorous check. One water supplier to South London, the Lambeth Water company, improved the quality of its product. It moved its source upstream so that the water stayed relatively free of sewage. Another supplier, the Southwark and Vauxhall Water Company, made no such change. The neighborhoods to the south of the river received a mix of water from the two companies. Snow calculated the deaths in subdistricts receiving water from Southwark and Vauxhall only, from Lambeth only, and from both. During the outbreak in the fall of 1853, the death rates per 100,000 were 114 in the Southwark and Vauxhall areas, zero in the Lambeth areas, and 60 in the mixed areas.[94]

Critics could again say that subdistricts most affected by the disease may have differed in ways other than the source of water. They may be exposed to different smells, have different levels of crowding and poverty, or differ in unknown ways that spread the disease. Snow was not content with his ecological analysis. He went further, again demonstrating his dogged detective work, by examining the water source and disease presence in individual homes. The fact was that water companies in South London sometimes competed to supply water to the same neighborhoods, streets, and individual homes.

Here is how Snow described the natural experiment:

No fewer than three hundred thousand people of both sexes, of every age and occupation, and of every rank and station, from gentlefolks down to the very poor, were divided into two groups without their choice, and, in most cases, without their knowledge; one group being supplied with water containing the sewage of London, and, amongst it, whatever might have come from the cholera patients, the other group having water quite free from such impurity.[95]

Other than the source of water, the two groups likely differed little from one another. They would have lived on the same streets, dealt with the same problems of poor housing and overcrowding, and breathed the same air.

Snow asked for the addresses of persons dying of cholera in parts of the city where the water supplied by the two companies was intermingled. He noted with understatement how difficult it was to obtain data on both the disease and water supply of specific homes: "The inquiry was necessarily attended with a good deal of trouble."[96] He often had to go door-to-door to get the data he needed. Even then, many residents did not know the company that supplied their water. Some residents could not be found, having died or left the area to avoid the epidemic. As Nigel Paneth notes, the burdensome work required him to abandon his medical practice for weeks at a time and convince others to help him. "Snow personally visited the homes of 658 people who died of cholera, ascertaining the water supply to each house."[97]

Even going door-to-door was not enough. When residents did not know the source of their water, which was all too typical, Snow had to devise other means to find out. He discovered that a chemical test for chloride of sodium in the water could distinguish the source. He asked the occupants for a sample of water, wrote the address on a vial, and brought the vial of water home for analysis.[98]

The findings over four weeks of the epidemic in 1854 were clear.[99] Of the 334 deaths from cholera in the area of study, 286 occurred in houses supplied by the Southwark and Vauxhall Water

Company and only 14 in houses supplied by the Lambeth Water Company. The former made up 86 percent of the total and the latter 4 percent. The other deaths came from people who dipped a pail directly into the Thames (7 percent) or obtained water from a pump well or ditch (2 percent). For the final 1 percent, the source could not be determined, such as for people who died while traveling.

Could the size of the populations account for these stark differences? Snow also divided the deaths from cholera by the population of houses served by the companies. The deaths per 10,000 were 315 for houses served by the Southwark and Vauxhall Water Company and 37 for houses served by the Lambeth Water Company. By comparison, the rate was 59 for the rest of London.[100]

The amount of detail provided in Snow's book is remarkable and highlights his meticulous research. The appendix lists the specifics of each of the 334 deaths, as in the first two entries:

> At 34, Charlotte Street, on 29th July, a stock-maker, aged 29, "Asiatic cholera 18 hours." Lambeth.
> At 45, Gravel Lane, on 1st August, the widow of a farmer, aged 48, "cholera 12 hours." Southwark & Vauxhall.

The details could "afford any person who wishes it an opportunity of verifying the result." But the investigator would need to take care to "to find the house where the attack took place, for in many streets there are several houses having the same number."[101]

To strengthen the results of the natural experiment, Snow piled on more facts. He compared the cholera mortality in 1849 and 1854 for the same districts. Recall that in 1849, the Lambeth Water Company had not yet improved the quality of the water. The changes made by the company between the two periods should affect cholera deaths. Snow did not have the house-by-house data, but aggregate comparisons were telling. Only the subdistricts supplied by the Southwark and Vauxhall Water Company showed an increase in mortality, while the those supplied by the Lambeth Water Company showed a decrease.[102]

Addressing Objections

Snow could conclude that "[t]he above instances are probably sufficient to illustrate the widely-spread influence which the pollution of the drinking water exerts in the propagation of cholera."[103] Like a good scientist, he carefully recognized the gaps in his knowledge, but he nevertheless was well prepared to answer the many objections posed to his arguments.

Some admitted the influence of polluted water on cholera but said that this was a predisposing factor that made people vulnerable to the real source of the disease in the atmosphere. Snow responded that this hypothesis could not "explain why nearly all the persons drinking it should be attacked together, in cases where a pump-well or some other limited supply is polluted, while the population around experience no increase of the malady."[104] Besides, doctors could visit patients and breath the same air but leave without getting sick. And densely populated areas suffered more from the disease than sparsely populated areas, even though blowing winds would affect both areas the same.

Others raised questions about apparent oddities in the spread of the disease. Why doesn't everyone who drinks contaminated water die? Snow reasonably said that not all water has the same concentration of the poison.[105] Why is the disease worse in the summer? People boil their water for tea in the winter but not in the summer and therefore drink safer water in the winter. Why are men affected more in the early stages of the epidemic and women at later stages? Men are more likely to move about for work and come in contact with the disease, but later women catch the disease when taking care of victims at home and sharing food with them. Why are children more vulnerable than adults? They are more likely to drink water than tea.[106] Why do some occupations such as sailor, hawkers, tanners, and weavers have higher rates of cholera death than other occupations? Sailors and tanners work in water, sailors and hawkers move about where they are exposed to the disease, and weavers are crowded together at work.[107] How can the disease spread upriver if contaminated water flows down river? Travelers with the disease travel upriver, spreading the disease from one village to another.[108]

If maps, natural experiments, and a wealth of facts were not convincing, a telling and sad story about a water inspector may have swayed skeptics. After attacks of cholera in a town near Bath, it appeared that overflow from privies contaminated the water from wells. Tenants using the well complained.

> The owner went himself, and on looking at the water and smelling it, he said that he could perceive nothing the matter with it. He was asked if he would taste it, and he drank a glass of it. This occurred on a Wednesday; he went home, was taken ill with the cholera, and died on the Saturday following, there being no cholera in his own neighbourhood at the time.[109]

While only an anecdote, it's striking enough to make the facts and numbers seem all the more real.

Snow's arguments had another appeal. People could not avoid breathing air, but they could take some simple measures to prevent the spread of the disease. Those coming in direct contact with a patient should carefully and frequently wash their hands, never touch food before washing, and avoid water from places where drains and sewers empty. If in doubt, boil water before drinking. Food and supplies from outside should be washed or boiled if possible. Linens should be cleaned and used carefully. Sick people should be separated from others, and perhaps most obviously, defecation should be kept separate from food.

Bigger and more difficult changes would be needed as well so that people had access to a plentiful supply of safe water.[110] Most obviously, water companies needed to supply river water from places that were distant from sewers and waste discharge. Human waste needed to be kept far from water wells, and crowded conditions that spread the disease needed to be improved. Housing for vagrants and poor people should be made cleaner, safer, and less crowded, and sick people coming to the country by ship should be segregated until they recover.

Chadwick and other health officials, although well intentioned, advocated for flushing sewers into streams and rivers. They wanted to get sewage out of the neighborhoods without any concern that it might make its way back to the neighborhoods via drinking water. Snow shared some of the goals for improved sanitation but understandably gave priority to drinking water. He saw that efforts to remove cesspits and backyard sewers turned out to increase the disease. Not only did it spread the disease to the river, but flushing sewage away used a lot of water, which meant water in reservoirs had less time for the disease to settle to the bottom.[111]

Critics Come Around—Eventually

Despite the strength of Snow's evidence, getting experts to abandon long-held and widely shared beliefs proved difficult. As David Wootton says, Snow's work was "a breathtaking, an astonishing performance" that presented a test for Snow's contemporaries, "a test they failed."[112]

Paneth summarizes the hostile, sometime vicious response to Snow's work: "The Lancet pilloried him, Parliament saw him as obstructionist, and John Simon (the leading public health official in London) virtually plagiarized his water supply data, only to have it serve a miasmatic interpretation."[113] With few exceptions, even his friends would not support him. Through all this, Snow "maintained cordial personal relations" with his critics and continued to participate in meetings dominated by his critics.[114] Still confident in his opinions, he applied in 1856 for a French award of £1,200 for controlling cholera, but the award committee turned down his application.[115]

Edwin Chadwick vigorously campaigned against Snow's theory.[116] The National Board of Health found no reason to accept Snow's arguments. A team of doctors, chemists, microscopists, and meteorologists was appointed in 1854 by the British government to investigate the cholera epidemic. After careful inquiry, the experts rejected Snow's claim of the waterborne nature of cholera in favor of contagion by "a wandering ferment in the atmosphere."[117] The critics claimed that Snow focused too narrowly on the single cause of contaminated water.[118] Disease was too complex, had too many causes, to reduce it to contaminated water and personal contact. Besides, unpleasant smells in the air were easy to identify, and it made sense that something so obvious would, under long-term exposure, harm the body.[119] An unknown substance hidden in the water was harder to accept.

Unfortunately for Snow, experts at the time proved skilled at adapting the miasma theory in creative and complex ways to account for findings consistent with Snow's waterborne evidence. They could say that contaminated water was sometimes a cause but not the major cause. They could say that sewers spread the disease by releasing foul air near water sources, not by contaminating the water itself. They could say that underground burial sites near water sources released diseased air that Snow had confused with contaminated water.[120]

Critics also had trouble accepting Snow's dismissal of moralistic explanations for the high cholera deaths rates among the poor and indigent populations. They pointed to personal weakness, unclean living, and lack of ambition as contributing to disease. With the support of ministers, physicians could argue that drinking, overeating, and sexual excess weakened the body in ways that made it vulnerable to disease.[121] Snow never blamed the behavior of people living in poverty, instead focusing on the difficulties of obtaining clean water and avoiding contact with sick persons in crowded housing. With more attention to hand washing, distance from the sick, use of clean water, and safe disposal of contaminated water, the residents of poor neighborhoods could reduce their risk of disease even without major changes in their living conditions.

One Dr. William Budd bravely came to Snow's defense. He found microscopic objects in the stools of cholera victims that he thought caused the disease and matched Snow's arguments. However, the Royal College of Physicians concluded that the microscopic objects were not the disease—they were skin cells and undigested food particles.[122] To be fair, the limited understanding of microbiology at the time left room for skepticism. Recognizing how little was known about cholera, some caution was warranted.[123]

Over the years, however, critics came to accept Snow's views. Two in particular who were initially skeptical of Snow's arguments would, through careful study, ultimately confirm them. One, a well-known and skilled statistical expert, used numbers. The other, a local cleric, interviewed the Soho residents affected by the epidemic.

The Statistician

William Farr has been called "probably the most important 19th century epidemiologist-statistician."[124] A physician with a good deal of skill with numbers, he obtained a job in the General Register Office related to censuses, vital statistics, and medical records. He eventually became the superintendent of the statistical department in the organization.[125] As superintendent, Farr provided Snow with data to analyze and the names and addresses of cholera victims to investigate. However, he initially did not share Snow's views on the cause of the illness. Like other experts, he explained the cholera outbreaks in 1848 and 1854 with his own version of the miasma theory.

Farr gathered figures for London neighborhoods on cholera death rates and on a variety of characteristics such as the density of the housing, the poverty of the residents, and the geography of the land. Crunching the numbers, he concluded that one key factor best explained the variation in cholera death rates across the neighborhoods—the elevation of the land above sea level. Low-lying London neighborhoods, typically alongside the Thames, had high death rates, while more elevated neighborhoods on hills farther from the river had low death rates.

The finding about the central role of elevation was fully consistent with the miasma theory. In low-lying areas, the harm of airborne disease particles was exacerbated by heavy, stagnant air and stable pools of rotting organic material. In elevated areas, breezes blew diseased air away, and the water flowing downhill would wash away disease-causing rotting material to low-lying areas. Elevation could explain the spread of cholera in the low-lying areas south of Thames and the low prevalence of the disease in the higher areas north of the Thames. Farr recommended measures to "prevent the formation of heavy mists or clouds of miasmatic material."[126]

Snow responded that elevation was spuriously related to mortality through water quality. Stagnant water in low-lying areas was more likely to be contaminated by discharges from diseased persons than water flowing more freely in high-lying areas. Besides, Snow could point out exceptions to the statistical association. Some high-lying areas suffered from the disease because of a contaminated water source, and some low-lying areas stayed relatively free from the disease because of a clean source of water.[127]

Farr eventually came to accept Snow's theory, although without abandoning his own ideas about the importance of elevation.[128] By 1866, some eleven years after Snow's book, new evidence from the most recent outbreak revealed a clear connection between the water supply and cholera deaths in East London. Farr came to advocate for Snow's claims, while suggesting that they were congruent with his own theory.

The Reverend

The Reverend Henry Whitehead had a personal interest in cholera. After ordination as a priest in the Anglican church, he took up his first position in 1851 at St. Luke's Church in Soho. A friendly figure among his Soho parishioners, Whitehead knew many of the victims of the 1854 outbreak. He wrote a short, seventeen-page pamphlet that year giving an eye-witness account of the deaths among his congregation.[129] He hoped that the document would dispel exaggerated and negative stories in newspapers, some of which said that hundreds lay dead in the streets of Soho.

Whitehead avoided any effort to identify the cause of the disease. The pamphlet made no mention of Snow's work, the Broad Street pump, or drinking water. In fact, he doubted the hypothesis. He recalled drinking water from the pump one night along with his brandy and being unaffected.[130] Later, in 1855, Whitehead read Snow's book but was not convinced, and he wrote to Snow to tell him so.[131] He reasoned that, with his knowledge of Soho and its people, he was in a position to carry out a study that would disprove Snow.[132]

Despite having no expertise in science or medicine, Whitehead proved to be an exceptional researcher. He visited the homes of

Soho residents who had died of cholera to get the facts on the timing of the fatal attacks, the sanitary conditions of their homes, and the consumption of water from the pump.[133] He was careful in his observations, precise in his measurements, and objective in his conclusions. "His tireless, repeated visits to the homes of the victims in his parish" exemplified the "shoe leather epidemiology" of Snow.[134]

Whitehead published his findings in June 1855 in a report, *Special Investigation of Broad Street*. "Slowly and I may add reluctantly," he concluded that the use of water from the Broad Street pump was connected to the epidemic.[135] For example, he described what happened in fifteen households with a cholera death.[136] Every case had a connection to the pump. He also confirmed a claim made by Snow about the death from cholera of the Hampstead widow living some distance from Soho. The widow's sons told Whitehead that she had shipped water from the Broad Street pump to her home. Although a layman, his thorough research impressed others. After seeing Whitehead's report, the Medical Committee of the General Board of Health concluded that the outbreak during August and September 1854 "was in some manner attributable to the use of the impure water of the well in Broad Street."[137]

With his research, Whitehead became a devoted admirer of Snow. Years later he would keep a portrait of Snow in his study. It remined him of the importance of the "patient study of the eternal laws."[138] He considered Snow to be "as great a benefactor . . . to the human race as has appeared in the present century."[139] According to Whitehead, Snow said, "You and I may not live to see the day, and my name may be forgotten when it comes, but the time will arrive when great outbreaks of cholera will be things of the past; and it is the knowledge of the way in which the disease is propagated which will cause them to disappear."[140]

Face-Off with Government Critics

Snow's single-minded devotion to his evidence in the face of hostility showed most clearly in an 1855 hearing before a parliamentary select committee involving a dispute between business owners and public health officials. The public health experts represented by members of the parliamentary committee accepted the miasma theory of contagion. If bad smells indicated the presence of disease in the air, it made sense to remove businesses that produced bad smells. Butchers, tanners, and soap makers all produced nasty odors. More than a nuisance, these smells were seen as a threat to public health. A bill in Parliament, the Nuisances Removal and Diseases Prevention Amendments Bill, would allow local governments to stop the release of malodorous fumes from certain types of businesses related to making soap and boiling animal parts.[141]

Naturally, the owners strongly opposed the bill—it would likely put them out of business. They sought out John Snow for support. The battle depended in good part on a question for medical science: To what extent did these industries spread disease in the city? Snow had no economic stake in the issues, but he had a strong opinion on the medical question. He agreed to serve as a witness for the business leaders and express his scientific views to Parliament.

In his testimony, Snow began by stating that the offensive trades targeted by the legislation did not contribute to the cholera epidemic. "In London, in any trade I am acquainted with, I do not believe that any decomposing vegetable or animal matters produce disease."[142] As evidence, he noted that the workmen involved in the trades did not suffer disproportionately from the disease. If the smells did not harm the workers in the immediate area, how could the flow of the disease through the air affect others far away? The workers and others living nearby might find the smells to be disgusting, but they were not at risk of cholera.

Members of the parliamentary committee were skeptical, even hostile of Snow's claims. One asked, "Have you never known the blood poisoned by inhaling putrid matter?" No, Snow responded. Extremely contaminated air might harm someone at the moment, but it does not result in a fever or lasting disease. A follow-up from a Mr. Egerton asked, "You mean to say, that the fact of breathing air which is tainted by decomposing matter, either animal or vegetable, will not be highly prejudicial to health?" Snow said, "I am not aware that it is." But haven't dead bodies poisoned people? Wouldn't the rotting flesh of a dead horse affect people nearby? "Yes, when those gases are extremely concentrated, they will actually poison a person and cause death, but not cause disease; those poisons do not reproduce themselves in the constitution."

Snow offered his alternative understanding of the disease. "I have satisfied myself completely, that the chief mode of propagation of cholera . . . was by the water of the Southwark and Vauxhall Water Company containing the sewage of London." It was also spread by human contact, particularly in crowded living conditions. It went from individual to individual, often family members, when one person accidentally swallowed what came from a sick person.

Committee members remained disbelieving. "Do you dispute the fact that putrid fever and typhus fever hang about places where there are open sewers?" Snow agreed that it occurs sometimes but that it was a coincidence. People congregate in places with open sewers and can communicate the disease to one another. Also, the water of pump wells is very often "impregnated with the excrements of the people, which soaks into the wells."

Still not convinced, their questions again pushed hard on the role of the offensive trades. Snow refused to qualify his claims: "I have every reason to believe that those trades have not had any influence whatever." One member responded, "Is it not possible that the same poisonous qualities which affect the water may be floating in the air?" Snow said that might be the case, but even so, any disease in the air must be swallowed in water or gotten directly from another person in the room.

The *Lancet*, a persistent critic of Snow and in favor of removing the offensive industries, was outraged. A comment on the testimony claimed that Snow offered no proof. He had only a theory "to the effect that animal matters are only injurious when swallowed!" It added that, "In riding his hobby very hard, he has fallen down through a gully-hole and has never since been able to get out again."[143] It made no sense to the author that swallowing water would cause disease while breathing gases would not. Nonetheless, Snow's testimony must have had some influence. The bill was changed in ways favorable to the manufacturers before being passed and becoming law.

The Making of a Public Health Hero

Sadly, Snow died relatively young, at age forty-five, in 1858. He fell off his chair and appeared to have suffered a stroke while working on his next book, *On Chloroform*.[144] Hoping to recover on his own, he rested, but after he vomited blood and became delirious at times, doctors were called. He lingered for five days before dying. An autopsy found shrunken and encrusted kidneys and listed kidney disease as an underlying contributor to his death. The kidney disease likely raised his blood pressure and led to the stroke.[145]

Snow in his last years had become a bit more sociable. He visited the opera on occasion, was known to tell funny stories, and admitted to some regret over not marrying.[146] But he was remembered after his death for his intellectual gifts. His friend Benjamin Richardson described Snow's strengths:

He had a patience that was inexhaustible, a devotion for labour unsurpassed, and a slow but sure and reliant comprehension and comprehensiveness which were not easily seen because of their extent. He combined with a stolid firmness distinctively Saxon a rare talent for penetration into obscure problems, for casting aside objects which are coincident or accidental, and for seizing determinately the realities for which he sought.[147]

The *Lancet* insultingly offered the two-line obituary that ignored his studies of cholera. Others, however, were more generous in submitting letters to the journal. One Dr. Hooper Attree said, "Who does not remember his frankness, his cordiality, his honesty, the absence of all disguise or affectation under an apparent off-hand manner? Her Majesty the Queen has been deprived of the future valuable services of a trustworthy, well-deserving, much-esteemed subject, by his sudden death."[148] A medical officer for a Soho workhouse, John French, confidently predicted "that the facts which have been brought to light by his indefatigable industry will prove to posterity that he was by far the most important investigator of the subject of cholera who has yet appeared."[149]

It is telling that the year of his death was also the year of what Londoners called the Great Stink. The smell from waste pumped into the river Thames became nearly intolerable during that summer—politicians in the Houses of Parliament located along the river complained of the foul air.[150] But there was no outbreak of cholera that summer. Despite exposure to the smells that many thought spread disease, improvements in the quality of drinking water had appeared to prevent a new outbreak. The Great Stink marked the start of the demise of the miasma theory.[151]

In response to the Great Stink, London committed to developing a network of sewers that would clean up the Thames. The engineer in charge, Sir Joseph William Bazalgette, designed a system with pumping stations that sent sewage downstream to be released at high tide, away from the city and into the sea. It took decades to complete the project, but along the way, it substantially reduced the risks of cholera. The next and last serious London outbreak of cholera in 1866 led to relatively few deaths, mostly isolated in a part of town where the new sewer system had not yet been extended.[152]

The benefits of water improvement vindicated Snow. In 1866, near the end of the last cholera epidemic in London, the *Lancet* finally gave Snow his due. In flowery language, an article in the journal proclaimed,

> We owe to him chiefly the severe induction by which the influence of the poisoning of water-supplies was proved. No greater service could be rendered to humanity than this; it has enabled us to meet and combat the disease, where alone it is to be vanquished, in its sources or channels of propagation. . . . Dr. Snow was a great public benefactor, and the benefits which he conferred must be fresh in the minds of all.[153]

The discoveries that ultimately proved Snow right also eclipsed his stature. Snow posited the existence of some kind of microorganism that caused cholera, but science at the time lacked the knowledge and technology to say more. The development of germ theory by Louis Pasteur in the early 1860s made Snow's ideas plausible.[154] The isolation of the *Vibrio cholerae* bacteria in 1884 by Robert Koch ultimately proved Snow correct.[155] With the advent of the new science of bacteriology, the battle against infectious disease moved away from Snow's methods, and his discoveries were largely forgotten.[156]

It was not until later in the twentieth century that awareness of Snow's work began to reemerge. In 1936, Wade Hampton Frost, a faculty member of the Johns Hopkins School of Hygiene and Public Health and the nation's first professor of epidemiology, wrote an introduction to the republication of *On the Mode of Communication of Cholera*. Frost viewed Snow's work as an exemplar for the new field.[157] Since then, the use of mapping, natural experiments, and statistical comparisons—all exemplified in Snow's studies—have become central to modern epidemiology. He is commonly referred to as the father of epidemiology.[158]

More important than the use of particular techniques was the strategy Snow applied to understand the mode of communication of disease.[159] Even without knowing the underlying cause of cholera, he posited a theory of disease transmission, drew out predictions based on the theory, and tested the predictions on human populations.[160] The findings led to community action and public policies to protect people, including cleaning up rivers, improving the quality of drinking water, and more safely disposing of human waste. Today, an army of scientists, researchers, and government officials across the world do the same to protect the safety of water.

As a result of public health efforts to prevent cholera, the disease has largely disappeared from high-income countries. It still emerges in lower-income countries, however, usually after some kind of disaster. Epidemics occurred in South America in 1991–1993 owing to poor-quality drinking water, in Haiti in 2010 after an earthquake, and in Yemen in 2017 during a period of civil war. The World Health Organization estimates 21,000 to 143,000 cholera deaths occur worldwide each year.[161] The problem persists not because we don't understand the disease agent but because of the failure of authorities to protect the water supply. Tracing the source of outbreaks today requires public health methods that, although more developed than those Snow used, continue to involve detective work based on data from human populations.

The crucial role of public health and the methods of John Snow have emerged in obvious ways during the recent COVID-19 crisis. While researchers develop vaccines, physicians experiment with treatments, and scientists seek to understand the nature of the virus, officials use public health methods to prevent the spread of the disease. They track who does and does not get the disease, search for patterns of communication, and recommend policies to minimize the threat. With regard to COVID-19, experts today are in a position similar to Snow's. They gain insight by measuring when, where, and among whom it spreads.

3.

The Progressive Chemist
Harvey Wiley and Food Safety

In 1902, twelve men joined an experiment that provided them with all their meals. They sat down in a basement room in the Department of Agriculture building to enjoy meals prepared by an accomplished chef. "The menu was wide and varied, and the chef, known only as 'Perry,' had an impressive resume. . . . The chicken was fresh, the potatoes perfectly prepared, the asparagus toothsome yet not tough. Everything was of the highest quality."[1] There was only one drawback—the food was mixed with poison.

The initial group of men, all volunteers, were healthy civil servants who had agreed to be part of a scientific experiment for one year and to not eat food outside the study dining room. As part of the experiment they were continuously inspected, probed, and tested to note any changes in their pulse, weight, or breathing. Their sweat, urine, and stools were collected and analyzed, and weekly physicals checked for any symptoms of disease or poor health. A photo of the participants (see page 111) shows a group of serious looking but mostly young and handsome men

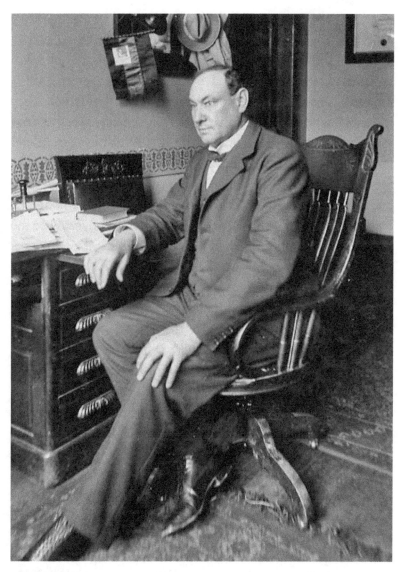

Harvey Wiley, 1900. *Source*: Wikimedia Commons, from DC Public Library
Commons.

wearing ties, dark suits, and high-collared white shirts.[2] They could pass for junior members of a prestigious law firm.

Initially, the cooks, under close supervision, mixed small amounts of poison into the food, but the men could detect changes in taste and avoided the poisoned items.[3] It was decided that they should instead take a gelatin capsule with their meals that contained the poison. This seemed to work well, as the capsules did not cause any immediate discomfort. The men did not object—they knew what the experiment involved when they joined. They understood the importance of determining if small amounts of poison caused long-term harm to health. More annoying were the constant examinations they underwent and the unpleasant task of collecting their own urine and feces.[4]

Once reporters found out about the experiment, they wasted no time in sensationalizing the story. A young reporter named George Rothwell Brown first used the name "Poison Squad" to describe the experimental subjects.[5] Reporters sought to interview the subjects, even asking questions through building windows. Restricting information about the experiment backfired, as reporters filled in gaps with rumors and speculation.[6] The experiment became so famous that poems and songs memorialized the squad.

Why would such an experiment be necessary? Isn't it obvious that poisoning food would be dangerous? On the contrary, many claimed that it was healthful. Food producers and sellers had found that adding small amounts of poisonous materials made foods cheaper, longer lasting, and more appetizing by maintaining their freshness and appearance. These preservatives prevented decay and spoilage in foodstuffs for long periods, allowing enough time to transport the products, store them in warehouses, display them on store shelves, and keep them in homes until ready for use. Advocates would say that small amounts of the poisons brought few risks relative to the advantages of production efficiencies and lower prices.

Take borax or boric acid, for example. It is a toxic substance that when ingested or inhaled will damage tissue, harm organs, and in large doses lead to death. As has been known for some time, these characteristics make borax an effective insecticide, one still used today. In food, borax prevents yeast, mold, and mildew from growing. It even improves the appearance of many foods, one reason for its common use in butter in the 1800s. These benefits, according to advocates, clearly outweighed the miniscule risks of the small amounts added to foods.

The man behind the experiment, Harvey Washington Wiley, chief chemist at the US Department of Agriculture, disagreed. He might have felt conflicted about feeding poison to his subjects. Even if the men willingly volunteered for the study and knew the risks, intentionally harming them might have seemed unethical. Yet, Wiley appears to have had little compunction about the experiment. Part scientist and part crusader, Wiley had dual motivations. As a chemist devoted to the scientific method, he wanted objective evidence on the harm of small doses of poisonous substances known to kill people in large doses. He had no doubt, but an experiment would offer proof. As an energetic crusader for the health of the public and an opponent of the businesses and industries that he accused of focusing only on profit, he wanted to convince the public and legislators that something needed to be done to protect consumers. An experiment would be persuasive.

Harvey Wiley was a strong-willed man. With what many saw as excessive single-mindedness, he fought for pure, unadulterated food in the United States. He was the motivating force behind passage in 1906 of the Pure Food and Drug Act, the legislation that eventually led to the US Food and Drug Administration. He offended many, including his bosses at the Department of

Agriculture and President Teddy Roosevelt, and he made power-ful enemies. His opponents found him to be a clever bureaucratic infighter and good at cultivating allies inside and outside the government. The public knew him as the famous Doc Wiley.[7]

The battle for food safety was fought on multiple fronts. It in-volved chemists in England who first documented the unhealthy adulteration of food in the early 1800s. It involved Louis Pasteur and the process of pasteurization to ensure the purity of milk and other products prone to carry bacteria. It involved public health advocates who objected to adding artificial chemicals and dis-tasteful substances to foods. And it involved early legislation in Great Britain in 1860 that first addressed food purity. All these ef-forts are important to the story of food safety.

But Harvey Wiley stands out. His status derived not just from his fame for the Poison Squad experiment, his fifty years of advocacy, or his role in passage of the Pure Food and Drug Act of 1906. Equally special was his strategy in campaigning for public health. He cultivated grassroots support for public health goals, most notably from women's groups. The widespread public an-ger over contaminated foods stirred by Wiley and others helped force unwilling politicians to respond to the demand for purer foods. His success illustrates the value of political pressure in translating scientific research into public health goals.

The task of mobilizing community action for public health pre-sented a particular challenge in the United States. Under the fed-eral system, the states had the power to regulate business, which complicated efforts to implement national food standards. Legis-lative action came more easily in Britain, where Parliament was the undisputed source of legislation on food safety. In the United States, it took someone with the stature, single-mindedness, and readiness for political battle of Harvey Wiley to bring about change. The results have over the long run led to one of the major achievements of public health—safer and healthier foods.[8]

The Problem with Food

Like sanitation and water quality, food emerged as a major public health problem as new industries and jobs attracted huge numbers of people to cities. The problem was simple: the populations of cities grew faster than the amount of food that nearby farmers and producers could supply. As buildings replaced fields and pastures in cities, food had to be shipped for greater distances to get to city residents. With longer and more complex supply chains, perishable foods—milk, meat, produce—could spoil, become contaminated, and lose their taste before getting to consumers. Milk, for example, was prone to spoilage and infection by dangerous bacteria.[9] Shipping by railroad into cities could speed the transportation of milk, but without refrigeration, its safety and quality suffered.

Sellers faced difficult choices. They could take precautions to protect the safety and quality of the food they sold, but such efforts raised the price beyond what most buyers could pay. Or they could maintain profit margins by enhancing the appearance and shelf life of their products but while also degrading the safety and quality of the food. All too often, they made the latter choice, and advances in science and chemistry helped them. By the 1800s, newly available chemicals could be added to foods, often at low prices. Many complained about such adulteration, but food laws were vague, and violations were difficult to prove.

Friedrich Accum

Laws would remain vague for some time to come, but proof of the widespread practice of adulterating food came in 1820 from a German chemist who lived in London as a young man. Friedrich Accum studied chemistry in his native Germany before moving to London in 1793 to work as a pharmacist.[10] In 1800, he set up a shop and laboratory in Soho—about an eight-minute walk from the location of the Broad Street pump that John Snow would make famous some years later. He developed skills in chemical analysis that, when combined with a showman's flair, made him a popular lecturer on chemistry.[11]

Accum was impressively productive. Books such as *System of Theoretical and Practical Chemistry* (published in 1803) and *A Practical Essay on the Analysis of Minerals* (published in 1804) plus dozens of scientific articles established his reputation. But one of his works stands out. In 1820, he published a book with a long-winded title that summarized its theme: *A Treatise on Adulterations of Food and Culinary Poisons: Exhibiting the Fraudulent Sophistications of Bread, Beer, Wine, Spirituous Liquors, Tea, Coffee, Cream, Confectionery, Vinegar, Mustard, Pepper, Cheese, Olive Oil, Pickles, and Other Articles Employed in Domestic Economy, and Methods of Detecting Them.* The book sold quickly, requiring a second edition in the same year. It popularly became known by the biblical quote adorning the cover. The words "There is death in the pot," are engraved on a serving vessel that contains a skull and whose decorative handles consist of two long, venomous snakes.

Right from the start, Accum warned readers about the dangers of the food they ate. He wanted to put the unwary on guard against ingenious methods of counterfeiting and adulterating food.[12] Sometimes these practices cheated buyers out of their money by substituting fake ingredients, but other times they poisoned consumers. All this was done, according to Accum, for "the eager and insatiable thirst for gain" of unprincipled dealers in victuals.[13] He wrote that "it would be difficult to mention a single article of food which is not to be met with in an adulterated state."[14]

The 360-page book covered hundreds of foods and their adulteration. The topics ranged from the obscure—exotic products such as Peruvian bark and rhubarb powder—to heavily consumed products such wine, bread, milk, coffee, pepper, tea, vinegar, beer,

A TREATISE

ON

ADULTERATIONS OF FOOD,

AND

Culinary Poisons,

EXHIBITING

THE FRAUDULENT SOPHISTICATIONS

OF

BREAD, BEER, WINE, SPIRITUOUS LIQUORS, TEA, COFFEE,

Cream, Confectionery, Vinegar, Mustard, Pepper, Cheese, Olive Oil, Pickles,

AND OTHER ARTICLES EMPLOYED IN DOMESTIC ECONOMY.

AND

Methods of detecting them.

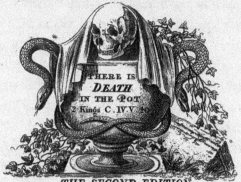

THERE IS
DEATH
IN THE POT
2 Kings C. IV. V.

THE SECOND EDITION.

BY FREDRICK ACCUM,

Operative Chemist, Lecturer on Practical Chemistry, Mineralogy, and on Chemistry
applied to the Arts and Manufactures; Member of the Royal Irish Academy
Fellow of the Linnæan Society; Member of the Royal Academy of
Sciences, and of the Royal Society of Arts of Berlin, &c. &c.

London:

SOLD BY LONGMAN, HURST, REES, ORME, AND BROWN,
PATERNOSTER ROW.

1820.

Cover of Friedrich Accum's *A Treatise on Adulterations of Food and Culinary Poisons*, 1820. *Source*: Wikimedia Commons, from Wellcome Images of Wellcome Trust. Creative Commons CC BY 4.0.

brandy, rum, and gin. All were adulterated in one form or another. Sometimes sellers mixed or replaced real products with counterfeit products, such as blending ground peas into coffee or replacing tea leaves with leaves from other plants. Poisonous substances were sometimes used to make foods appear more appetizing. For example, brewers used the extract from a poisonous root to save on the cost of malt and hops used in beer. Wine sellers added lead to make white wine transparent, and gin included substances such as lead and alum.[15] Although small, the quantities could slowly poison drinkers.

The book was a worldwide success and marked the start of a pure food movement.[16] The book's popularity earned it enemies, however. It listed food producers and sellers by name and threatened the livelihood of many businesses. Soon after publishing the book, Accum was forced to leave England and return to Germany. He was accused of ripping pages from books at the Royal Institution in London rather than copying them by hand.[17] Although no evidence exists of a conspiracy by his opponents to prosecute him, the timing is suspicious. He returned to Germany, quietly serving out the rest of his life as a professor in Berlin.

Others followed up on Accum's work. Thomas Wakley, editor of the *Lancet* (and, incidentally, a critic of John Snow), became a crusader for safer food. Arthur Hassall, hired by Wakley, provided more scientific evidence of adulteration, and John Postgate, a surgeon, lobbied Parliament to pass a law preventing adulteration of food.[18] In 1860, Parliament enacted the first nationwide law, the Adulteration Act. Generally considered a failure, the law was criticized for its ambiguous definition of adulteration and its reliance on poor-quality chemical analyses.[19] The 1860 law was followed by the 1875 Sale of Food and Drug Act, which proved to be more lasting and effective.[20] The law was nonetheless only the start of uneven enforcement efforts to make food safer.

Swill Milk

In 1858, a newspaper editorial called out "murderers" who distributed "liquid poison" in New York City. The angry writer went on: "For the midnight assassin, we have the rope and the gallows; for the robber the penitentiary; but for those who murder our children by the thousands we have neither reprobation nor punishment. They are not penal villains, but licensed traders, and though their traffic is literally in human life the Government seems powerless or unwilling to interfere."[21] The deadly poison was the milk sold throughout the city; the villains were the producers and sellers. The complaints about milk quality and the helplessness of consumers to control it made the product a target in the battle for food safety. Milk had importance both for its popularity and propensity to spoil and carry dangerous bacteria.

Milk in New York City and other large towns at the time was indeed shockingly bad. Although labeled "Pure Country Milk," the product often came from cows located in nearby city stables that were filthy enough to turn the stomach of observers. Without pastureland or even spacious stables, the cows were crowded together in unhealthy conditions. Equally bad, they were fed swill—the hot grains left over from distilling alcohol. The fermentation process removed the starch and alcohol from the grain, leaving slop with little nutritional value.[22] So common was the practice that stables were often located next to distilleries.

The "swill milk" from the cows was a sickly, bluish color. "To mask this ghastly color, the distilleries added chalk, eggs, flour, water, molasses, and other substances."[23] Dairymen further profited from skimming off cream and watering down what was left. As Deborah Blum summarizes, "The standard recipe was a pint of lukewarm water to every quart of milk—after the cream had been skimmed off. To improve the bluish look of the remaining liquid, milk producers learned to add whitening agents such as plaster of paris or chalk."[24] So common was watered-down milk in poor districts "that the local water pump was commonly referred to as 'the cow's second tail.'"[25] Some additives were a threat to health. To preserve the milk and prevent it from souring, producers would add boric acid and formaldehyde, both poisons.[26] Chemical preservatives were given names such as Preservaline, Freezine, and Freezem to hide the real ingredients, namely, salicylic acid, sodium sulfite, and formaldehyde.[27]

Concern about milk stemmed from more than adulteration and poor nutritional quality. More worrying were the diseases it carried. City dairies were unhygienic places. Milkers and milk pails were dirty, fecal matter from the cows could get in the milk, and unsafe storage allowed bacteria to grow. Until bottles were used regularly, milk was distributed haphazardly in pails open to whatever might fall in.[28]

Many suspected that milk spread diseases such as scarlet fever, diphtheria, typhoid, and tuberculosis. Tuberculosis was a special concern, as Robert Koch had shown that one strain of the germ was spread from cows to people via milk.[29] We know today that milk can "carry dangerous bacteria such as *Salmonella, E. coli, Listeria, Campylobacter*, and others that cause foodborne illness."[30] The problem became all the more serious in the 1800s. As Mark Kurlansky points out, "In the 18th and 19th centuries, as drinking milk became more fashionable, Europeans and Americans increasingly turned away from breastfeeding and wet nursing and toward artificial feeding."[31] The high demand for milk combined with its poor quality caused a rise in infant deaths.[32]

The means to protect milk from bacteria had been recognized, if not understood, for some time. Boiling food had been found to preserve it for longer periods. In the early 1800s, methods were developed to boil bottled foods and create canned goods. Proof of the benefits came in 1864 from Louis Pasteur. In his studies of fermentation, he laid the groundwork for the discovery of bacteria as living organisms. As a practical application, he found that heating wine to between 122 and 140 degrees Fahrenheit killed microbes in the wine, after which it could be safely left to age. In honor of his discovery, the heating process was named "pasteurization." Yet, even with its well-established benefits, milk would not be regularly subjected to pasteurization until decades later. In the meantime, drinking contaminated milk continued to spread disease.

From Log Cabin to Government Expert

It's hard to know what made Harvey Wiley so stubbornly persistent, so willing to fight battles with his bosses, Congress, powerful business interests, and even the president of the United States. No doubt he was motivated by the importance of the issue of food safety. He wanted to help people, to improve the health of the public. But he also had a personality and upbringing that suited him well for the battles to come.

A Strong Sense of Right and Wrong

Harvey Washington Wiley was born in a log cabin in 1844, the son of Indiana farmers. In the days before high-end tractors and mechanical harvesters, work on the farm depended on the physical labor of family members. He helped to plant and harvest crops, tapped maple trees to prepare syrup and sugar, and completed the daily chores required on a farm.[33] Perhaps in part from the physical labor, he had in his own words, "a tall robust physique."[34] The chores no doubt encouraged discipline and effort. A hard worker at school as well as at home, he spent hours in the school library. He developed an early interest in chemistry as a young man, an interest that he would maintain for the rest of his life.[35]

Wiley's father was deeply religious, serving as a lay preacher. He taught his son the importance of doing right, even when unpopular. The dominant issue of the time, slavery, divided free states like Indiana. His father vigorously opposed slavery, even helping runaway enslaved people on the underground railroad. Wiley similarly felt bitter antagonism toward the institution.[36] As a young man, he joined the Union Army to fight for this righteous cause, although sickness prevented him from seeing combat.[37]

After the war, he finished his undergraduate degree at Hanover College, an experience he describes with warmth and gratitude in his autobiography. Immediately after his graduation ceremony, he returned to his parents' farm to spend the summer working in the fields. By then he had decided to study medicine but needed a way to pay for the training. He accepted a teaching job in Indiana and was thrilled to receive his first wages ever—$60 a month.[38] After beginning his medical studies in 1868, by working with a country doctor of his acquaintance, he received an offer to teach Latin and Greek at Northwestern Christian University in Indianapolis, where he could also study at a new medical school in the city.[39]

He said that he was so devoted to his professional accomplishments at the time that he was "perfectly immune to any serious affairs of the heart."[40] Apparently so, as his autobiography mentions no romance until late in life. Devoutly religious at the time, he often led prayers at the school. Otherwise, hard work dominated, and he received his MD degree from Indiana Medical College in 1871.[41]

Rather than practice as a physician, Wiley decided to teach school again but soon went to Harvard to attend lectures and receive a bachelor of science degree. Armed with his new degree, he returned to teaching chemistry at the Indiana Medical College.[42] During that time, he barely survived a severe case of cerebrospinal meningitis that left him unconscious for three weeks. Doctors wanted to amputate his leg, but he refused and surprisingly recovered fully.[43] Soon after, he accepted an offer to become a professor of chemistry at Purdue University.

Commitment to Food Science

At Purdue, he developed his interest in food science, even going to Germany in 1878 to study at the Imperial Health Office.[44] The work proved so compelling that he abandoned any plans to practice medicine.[45] He specialized in the chemistry of sugar—how it can be extracted from sugar cane and sugar beets and how it can be analyzed chemically.[46] The research sounds narrow and unexciting, but it placed him at the center of a controversy. The State Board of Health, having concerns about the adulteration of sugar, asked Wiley to examine sugars and syrups sold in the state. He found that glucose, a simple sugar that could be manufactured at low cost, had often been added to commercially sold honey, syrups, and molasses. Beekeepers viewed the criticism of honey as a threat to their industry, angrily calling claims of adulteration the "Wiley lie."[47] Wiley brought the beekeepers to his side, however, by arguing that he was protecting their legitimate honey from the unfair competition of counterfeit products.

Wiley appeared to be an engaging teacher and popular with students. Outside of class, he enjoyed playing baseball and football with students. One photo from his time at Purdue shows him wearing an old-fashioned helmet and holding a football.[48] When the president of Purdue stepped down, students started a campaign, much against Wiley's wishes, to appoint him to the newly opened position. He told them that he wanted to continue his work on food chemistry and adulteration.[49] The students continued their campaign, but to Wiley's relief, the board of trustees appointed someone else to the presidency.

Wiley diverged in other ways from the norm of professorial behavior. He was almost fired for riding a bicycle. As Wiley tells the story,

I acquired a bicycle uniform with knee breeches, and I rode daily through the streets of Lafayette, over the bridge across the Wabash and up to the university, frightening horses, attracting attention and grieving the hearts of the staid president and professors, as well as members of the board of trustees.[50]

So new was bicycle riding in the town that it shocked some at the university. One member of the board of trustees complained:

He has put on a uniform and played baseball with the boys, much to the discredit of the dignity of a professor. But the most grave offense of all has lately come to our attention. Professor Wiley has bought a bicycle. Imagine my feelings and those of other members of the board on seeing one of our professors dressed up like a monkey and astride a cart wheel riding along our streets.[51]

When brought before the board, Wiley offered his resignation, which was refused, but the harm was done.

His reputation had grown, and his contacts had widened to such a degree that, unexpectedly, he received an offer to become the chief of the Division of Chemistry (renamed the Bureau of Chemistry in 1901) of the US Department of Agriculture (USDA). Wiley's research on the chemistry of sugar made him a good choice in the view of USDA officials. They wanted someone to use science to improve the US sugar crop and reduce the need for imports.[52] His ties to Purdue had deteriorated with the bicycle incident and the inability to do much as a professor to guide public policies on food quality. During his nine years at Purdue, Wiley came to "believe that tremendous changes had to be brought about before there would be anything like the protection the public needed from impure and dangerous substances."[53] He decided to accept the position in Washington, DC.

He came to the nation's capital in June 1883 with the expectation that he would stay for the long-term.[54] He immediately faced trouble. The previous chief chemist, dismissed by the commissioner of agriculture after a dispute, sought to get his job back by disparaging Wiley as unsuited for the position. The public condemnations were unfair and hurtful.[55] Although unused to such treatment, Wiley found that replying to the attacks was "a poor way to answer such charges and that the best way is to go about one's business and let enemies do their worst."[56]

The experience foretold what would happen during Wiley's time at the Department of Agriculture. "I was in the midst of a continual fight from beginning to end; but always I did what I thought was right, forged ahead and usually won."[57] He had the right temperament for the fight. His co-workers called him a man of kind heart with a cordial, courageous personality,[58] while others viewed him as stubborn and self-righteous. As a young man, he had an impressive appearance, being tall and stocky with a jet-black beard, mustache, and hair. He had "a rough-hewn oval face, with a prominent nose and slanting black eyes remarkable for their penetrating glance."[59] A sociable, engaging personality earned him devoted friends and supporters to balance tendencies toward anger and arrogance. He was more personable than the bullying Edwin Chadwick and more sociable than the introverted John Snow. These traits plus immense energy and ambition made Wiley exceptional as both a friend and enemy.

The Progressive Era

Wiley was committed to the causes of the Progressive Era, a period from roughly the 1890s to the 1920s that saw widespread social activism and political and economic reform. The era was a response to some difficult decades of American life. The Civil War and the failure of Reconstruction to provide equal rights to African Americans had been followed by a period of rapid industrial growth that worsened the gap between owners and workers, natives and immigrants, and whites and Blacks. Businessmen and financiers—called "robber barons" by critics and "captains of industry" by supporters—benefited handsomely from the boom. Men such as John D. Rockefeller, Andrew Carnegie, and J. P. Morgan gained such astounding wealth and spent it so ostentatiously that Mark Twain called the period the Gilded Age. The showy wealth of the time looked like gold on the outside but covered ugly problems underneath—corruption, exploitation, poverty, and unethical business practices.

The excesses of the Gilded Age led to Progressive Era demands for more democratic and activist governments. An amazing variety of social movements during this period, many still with us today, gathered under the umbrella term of progressivism:

- The women's suffrage campaign led to the ratification in 1920 of the Nineteenth Amendment to the Constitution, which gave women the right to vote;
- new organizations such as the NAACP, founded by W. E. B. Du Bois and others in 1909, advocated for the rights of African Americans;
- reforms to professionalize municipal workers gave citizens a larger role in selecting political candidates and weakened the corrupt political machines in large cities;
- antitrust laws (or trust-busting) regulated monopolies and uncompetitive corporations; and
- temperance groups helped ratify the Eighteenth Amendment in 1919 to prohibit the manufacture, transportation, export, or sale of intoxicating liquor.

The cause of safe food meshed well with these progressive movements. Like those advocating for other causes, proponents of food safety called for fairer, more equal, and more democratic access to the government. They sought to protect the public from the corruption of food quality by greedy businessmen much as trustbusters sought to protect the public from unfair business practices, temperance leaders sought to protect families from the harm of alcohol, and reformers sought to give voters more say in city elections and policies. Governments served as the primary means to bring about such changes. Wiley embodied the ethos of the Progressive Era. He favored vigorous government regulation and was ahead of his time in his backing of equality for women and African Americans.

The person most associated with the progressive movement, Teddy Roosevelt, served as the twenty-sixth US president from 1901 to 1909. The youngest American president—he was forty-two years old when first assuming the office—Roosevelt is known for his support of civil service reform, antitrust actions, and federal legislation to ban impure food and drugs. Although so angered by Wiley that he once wanted him to be fired, Roosevelt was a key player in the fight for safe food.

The press had a leading role in the reforms of the Progressive Era. The period has been called the Golden Age of Journalism.[60] In exposing political corruption, fraudulent business practices, and the miseries of the poor, writers and reporters took on diffi-cult causes. Their vivid stories on mistreatment of the vulnerable by the well-off gained wide readership. Somewhat critically, Teddy Roosevelt used the term "muckraker" to describe these journal-ists. But their stories were vital to uncovering wrong-doing and mobilizing the public. Wiley, seeing the value of the press in his campaign for food safety, would take advantage of publicity from newspapers and magazines whenever he could.

One of the most famous muckrakers, Upton Sinclair, unintentionally became central in the campaign for food safety. More a poet and writer than journalist, Sinclair nonetheless has a prominent place among muckraking journalists for his 1906 book, *The Jungle*. The novel dramatized what Sinclair saw during seven weeks of undercover observations in Chicago meat-packing plants. It depicted the disgusting and unsanitary practices used in meat production and the exploitation of poor immigrants by the industry. Sinclair, who would run for Congress as a socialist, was dismayed that his readers focused on the filthy meat rather than the plight of the workers. But few could ignore the descriptions of blood, feces, and dirt on the floor, workers falling into rendering vats, and scooped-up dirt, rats, and poison from the floor being used to makes sausages. Despite dislike of Sinclair's socialism, Roosevelt saw the need for action after reading *The Jungle*. The book roused politicians and consumers who otherwise knew little about the routine adulteration of their food and drink.

In some ways, Wiley was seen as a muckraker.[61] His pronouncements about adulteration reflected his progressive views and could go beyond the chemical evidence.[62] The combination of science and passion would make him enemies as well as gain him supporters, but like muckrakers espousing other causes, his strategy worked.

At the USDA

Wiley began his new position in 1883, at the young age of thirty-eight. The opportunities to do something important did not look promising. He ran a tiny division with labs located in a damp and dark basement.[63] The stale air was bad enough that Wiley banned smoking. The Department of Agriculture, created only twenty-one years earlier in 1862 by President Lincoln, aimed primarily to help farmers produce and sell more crops. It seemed an unlikely center for an innovative movement to enhance the health of the public. Nevertheless, Wiley would stay in the position for the next twenty-nine years.

Wiley's efforts to improve food safety represented a shift in the approach to public health. Past advances focused on limiting the spread of infectious diseases. The movement for food safety, particularly as it related to milk, had a component of disease prevention as well—but of a different sort. Adulterated food could lead to a buildup of harmful chemicals in the body and chronic poor health rather than infection and acute sickness. The chemicals did not kill in a few days or weeks and, although harder to document, the damage was real. Preventing the harm required chemists and the chemical analysis of food.

The Battle for Federal Legislation Begins

Once settled in his new job, Wiley focused first on sugar but made little progress in replacing imports with native crops. All the while, he had to stay politically vigilant in protecting his division from new USDA bosses and new presidential administrations.[64] Although not successful in his sugar program, "he found salvation for his division and fame for himself in making the rising concern about food purity his own."[65] The issue resonated with Wiley's upbringing of eating local farm food and was compatible with his progressive mindset.

In 1889, Wiley obtained funds from Congress for the study of food adulteration.[66] It turned out that, much like Friedrich Accum, Wiley's background as a chemist would serve him well in investigating suspect food products. The staff of inspectors and analysts he hired shared his enthusiasm for the cause.[67]

A series of reports on food adulteration, *Bulletin 13 on Foods and Food Adulteration*, steadily emerged from the Chemistry Division from 1887 through 1907.[68] Studies found that food producers added benzoate of soda, alum, sulfurous acid, salicylic acid, and similar adulterants. Added copper gave canned vegetables a vivid green color. Sulfur dioxide was used to bleach sugar, and saccharine was used as a substitute for sugar to make foods sweeter.[69] Red lead was added to cayenne pepper, and metallic dyes made candies colorful.[70] In some cases, it was hard to know if these chemical additives were harmful to health, and debate continues today over the safe usage of some of them. Wiley was convinced they were harmful or at least of little benefit.

Even if adulterants were not harmful, manufacturers were deceiving consumers about what they were eating and drinking. Wiley accused distillers of adding colors and flavors to pure alcohol to imitate whiskey, brandy, and rum.[71] Other chemists studying adulteration found that coffee included "chicory, caramel, and numerous roasted grains, such as corn, wheat, and rye, as well as such roots and seeds as dandelion, mangold wurzel, turnips, beans, peas, etc."[72]

Another source of fraud that related to medicines rather than food nonetheless became part of the battle for food safety. Patent medicines that relied on outrageous promises, fake testimonials, and impressive-sounding names were sold commercially as self-treatments for a variety of ailments. Although quack remedies based on fraudulent claims had been around for centuries, patent medicines enjoyed a period of particular popularity during the late 1800s, largely because of misleading advertising. Wiley was more concerned with food but understood that sellers of these products preyed on the sick and vulnerable, falsely raising their hopes to be healed. The claims to cure asthma, bronchitis, bowel troubles, coughs, colds, cancers, tuberculosis, fever, influenza, dysentery, diarrhea, indigestion, malaria, skin disease, ulcers, and dandruff were as astounding as they were wrong. Investigations of the products by his unit made the fraud clear. For example, one patent medicine was found to consist of mostly water plus some sulfuric and sulfurous acids and hydrochloric and hydrobromic acids.[73]

At least initially, the bulletins on food adulteration published by the Chemistry Division had modest influence on the public. But they did get the attention of those who sold adulterated and counterfeit food and medicine. They disputed claims of fraud and physical harm from their products and often had allies in Congress and the press to help them. Critics called Wiley "the chief janitor and policeman of the people's insides."[74] One senator from New York ridiculed the idea of letting chemists at the Department of Agriculture tell people what to eat and drink.[75] Wiley did not back down in the face of opposition. To the contrary, "[f]aced with hostility, he became more rigid in his stance, often refusing to compromise even on small details.[76]

Along with angering opponents in business and industry, Wiley regularly upset his bosses at the Department of Agriculture. Julius Sterling Morton, secretary of agriculture from 1893 to 1897, sought to cut spending at the USDA and by the end of his term even recommended abolishing the department.[77] He opposed Wiley's studies of sugar, suspecting that Wiley used the experimental stations he had set up for personal gain. Morton even appointed a committee to investigate Wiley's financial dealings.[78] Despite some petty accusations about his misuse of funds, Wiley managed to hold on to his job until Morton left.

A more serious enemy was James Wilson, the secretary of agriculture from 1897 to 1913. Wilson initially supported the research on food adulteration but found that Wiley's ambitions often led to conflict with others. He thought that Wiley was getting "too big for his trousers."[79] Wilson had a point, as even admirers of Wiley noted, "His crusading nature endeared him to about half of the state food officials but alienated him from the other half."[80] Wilson eventually came to be part of the other half. Wiley in turn came to disagree with Wilson's policies. Describing Wilson, Wiley remarked that "he had the greatest capacity of any person I ever knew to take the wrong side of public questions, especially those relating to health through diet."[81]

Wiley even angered Theodore Roosevelt early in his presidency. As Wiley tells the story, Roosevelt wanted to import more sugar from Cuba, while Wiley had been working for decades in behalf of the American sugar industry, which would be hurt by the imports. In testifying before Congress about reducing the costs of importing sugar, he stated, "I consider it a very unwise piece of legislation and one which will damage, to a very serious extent, our domestic sugar industry."[82] After seeing headlines about the statement, Roosevelt demanded Wiley's resignation. The president relented on his demand, but tensions between the two would continue.

Grassroots Support

Not content to publish chemical analyses, Wiley advocated for legislative action to give responsibility for regulating food and drugs to the federal government. He testified often before Congress and developed strong ties to many members.[83] Time and again, however, proposed legislation failed to pass. "There seemed to be an understanding between the two Houses that when one passed a bill for the repression of food adulteration the other would see that it suffered a lingering death."[84]

Some states had passed their own laws to protect the purity and quality of food. Although steps in the right direction, the state laws were too scattered and inconsistent to be effective. The country needed encompassing federal laws. Unfortunately, many in Congress objected in principle to such federal legislation. They believed that food laws were the province of the states, as the Commerce Clause of the Constitution did not permit the federal government to regulate business nationwide. Supporters of the free market agreed, predicting that such legislation would harm the economy. And, of course, many food manufacturers and sellers vociferously opposed any legislation to regulate their products.

Wiley realized that working with Congress and federal agencies and publishing bulletins on food adulteration would not bring about the changes in food safety that he sought. If he could convince the public of the importance of the issue, pressure from constituents would then convince Congress to make changes. An effective campaign for food safety certainly needed a leader, and Wiley was well-suited for the task. His dark looks and imposing stature combined with a sense of humor, personal charm, and theatrical flair made him an impressive champion of the cause.[85] "He addressed civic organizations, trade associations, scientific societies, labor unions, church groups and committees of Congress with equal zest and effectiveness."[86] In so doing, he created a strange alliance of supportive businesses, state agricultural chemists, physicians, women's clubs, and journalists that became a potent pressure group.[87] The American Medical Association, while not a leader in the pure food movement, provided significant support to Wiley.[88] Even some businesses concerned about unfair competition and wanting to have a clear set of standards to follow committed to Wiley's campaign.[89]

Wiley found a particularly receptive audience among diverse women's groups across the country. He tirelessly encouraged them to join his campaign for national food safety legislation and worked closely with their leaders. "Like an itinerant preacher," he stumped across the country, treating every women's club as a pulpit.[90] Women were a receptive audience for his message. Given gender roles at the time, food purity was high among their concerns for home protection and child and family health. Stories of children who died from contaminated milk or became sick from adulterated food naturally frightened mothers. Even cookbook authors complained about the unhealthy pollution of commercial food.[91]

More generally, many women shared Wiley's progressive values favoring a democratically constituted and activist government that worked in behalf of the wider public rather than politicians and special interest groups. Denied the democratic right to vote, women felt the unfairness of the system with particular intensity. Women's groups worked broadly in support of many issues—child labor laws, relief for poor people, and prevention of alcohol abuse— but they had special authority on food issues. Men more willingly deferred to women on matters relating to home and family. Women were seen as less motivated by financial interests than men,[92] and they could legitimately organize under the banner of home purity.[93]

Despite not having the vote, women wielded considerable influence in the pure food movement. As one editorial at the time put it, "Now let the food adulterer quail, for we have the women on our side."[94] They could write letters, attend rallies and speeches, and pressure lawmakers. Such actions helped mobilize public opinion on a national scale. The strategy of building a mass grassroots movement rather than appealing to a small group of influential men was new but proved to be effective. Wiley himself credited women for turning the tide of public opinion in favor of pure food.[95]

A surprising but nonetheless important ally was the Woman's Christian Temperance Union. Although a religious organization primarily devoted to restricting or banning alcohol, the group had more wide-ranging concerns about harmful substances.[96] The adulteration of food, drink, and medicines with chemicals, alcohol, and drugs (at one time, Coca-Cola included cocaine) encouraged the kind of intemperance the organization opposed. These concerns led the organization to include pure food as part of its political activism.[97]

Wiley's respect for women activists and collaboration with women's organizations reflected a broader respect for women that was unusual for the times. Having three sisters who went to college and shared in the demands of farm work, Wiley viewed women as smart, strong, and capable.[98] Though far from a feminist—he once wrote that women were "not intended by nature, by taste, nor by education, as a rule, to follow the pursuits which are reserved for men"[99]—he encouraged their progressive activities.

The Poison Squad

Wiley had been living in Washington, DC, and fighting against food adulteration for some time before he devised the experiment that made him most famous. As a scientist, he wanted to learn if commonly used food preservatives were harmful and if so, was there a safety threshold below which no harm occurred. It would be important to separate fact from sensationalized scare stories and assertions of no risk. The ultimate goal was to provide evidence of harm that would justify a national policy to regulate food additives. If he "could prove from his studies that food adulteration went beyond flagrant cheating to obvious harm, then both the public and Congress would likely support a national policy."[100]

He convinced members of Congress in 1902 to fund the research.[101] Chemical preservatives were a logical choice for study. They were used widely, considered harmful in large doses, and claimed by manufacturers to be safe in small doses. Wiley initially decided to study five common food preservatives: borax, salicylic acid, sulfuric acid, sodium benzoate, and formaldehyde.[102] Other chemicals to be studied included potassium nitrate, copper sulphate, and saccharin.[103] The chemicals would be mixed with food in varying amounts before being served. A team of scientists would monitor changes in the health of the subjects.

Wiley found it surprisingly easy to recruit subjects. Young, healthy men from the Department of Agriculture and the Georgetown Medical College volunteered for the study. A group photo (with Harvey Wiley standing in the middle) conveys their youthfulness and seriousness. Over the full five years of the experiment, there was never trouble finding volunteers.[104] The men received free meals but had to eat them in the basement of the Agriculture Department building, located on what is now Independence Avenue. They could consume no outside foods or beverages, except water, and had to report any violations of the rules. For young men living alone, free and expertly prepared food was an attraction. After some problems with degradation of the taste of the foods by the additives, subjects merely had swallow gelatin capsules with the prescribed amount of the additive. The constant weight, temperature and pulse measurements were more of a chore.[105] Worse, they had to collect their urine, feces, and sweat for analysis.

Today, the men appear brave given the dangers and the modest rewards. They knew they could get sick, as they had to agree not to hold the government responsible for any harm or injury.[106] But Wiley sought to minimize any serious risks. He declared, "I allowed no experiment to be carried to the point of danger to health."[107] He would stop the experiments when "the chemicals made several of the diners so sick that they couldn't function—nausea, vomiting, stomachaches, and the inability to perform work of any kind."[108]

As word got out about the experiment, it not surprisingly attracted national attention. Wiley worried that, by treating the study as a source of humor or scare stories, the press would belittle the seriousness of the results. He tried to keep the subjects from talking to the press and said little himself. He eventually gave in after reporters managed to interview the chef through a basement window.[109] It would be better to answer questions directly.

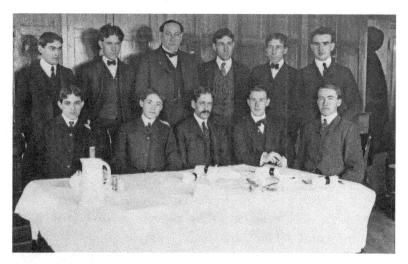

Harvey Wiley (*back row, third from left*) and his "Poison Squad." *Source*: Wikimedia Commons, from the US Food and Drug Administration.

The experiment, which lasted from 1902 to 1907, produced an enormous amount of data. Subjects receiving doses of borax reported discomfort, headaches, and inability to work, and subjects receiving doses of benzoate of soda lost weight and their appetite.[110] In Wiley's own summary of the results, "the lesson they taught was clear and unmistakable: preservatives used in foods are harmful to health."[111] He admitted that very small amounts of preservatives might be harmless and might be justified by the benefits of protecting consumers from the dangers of food spoilage. But he still believed that dangerous additives could accumulate in the body and that consumers could best be protected by applying clearly defined restrictions to all preservatives.[112]

The study lacked the strengths of double-blind trials with random assignment to intervention and control groups. Despite these faults, the results of the study and the publicity it generated helped pass new legislation. Four of the preservatives—borax, salicylic acid, formaldehyde, and copper sulfate—are no longer used.[113] As for the subjects, there is only anecdotal evidence that no one suffered long-term harm. William O. Robinson of Falls Church, Virginia, one of the subjects participating in the study, died in 1979 at age ninety-four. He said that no one suffered permanent illness or injury.[114]

Success and Conflict

The Laws

Spurred by the fame of *The Jungle*, exposés of fraudulent patent medicines, and the Poison Squad, Congress finally acted after having failed to pass the nearly one hundred bills that had been introduced since 1879.[115] With the support of President Roosevelt, who overcame his continued annoyance with Wiley, Congress passed two groundbreaking legislative acts in 1906 that regulated food and drugs at the national level. The two pieces of legislation stand out as landmarks of the Progressive Era in assigning responsibility for the health and safety of the public to the federal government. Although some states had their own laws, they were powerless to prevent distribution of adulterated products across state lines. The new laws aimed to solve that problem.

First, the Meat Inspection Act required that stockyards slaughter animals and butcher meat under sanitary conditions and made it illegal to sell misbranded or adulterated meat. The act had four key provisions: (1) mandatory inspection of livestock before slaughtering, (2) mandatory inspection of carcasses after slaughtering, (3) sanitary standards for slaughterhouses, and (4) inspection and enforcement by the Department of Agriculture. The law would guide the regulation of meat production for the next sixty years.

Second, the Pure Food and Drug Act prohibited "the addition of any ingredients that would substitute for the food, conceal damage, pose a health hazard, or constitute a filthy or decomposed substance. . . . Also, the food or drug label could not be false or misleading in any particular, and the presence and amount of eleven dangerous ingredients, including alcohol, heroin, and cocaine, had to be listed."[116] It required that drugs include a label with a list of active ingredients and meet certain purity standards. Importantly, Congress assigned inspection powers to the Bureau of Chemistry, which Wiley led.

As indicated by its name, the new law regulated drugs as well as food. It sought to protect the public from ineffective or harmful drugs. But rather than requiring proof that the drug worked as advertised, it mandated accurate product labeling. The drugs needed to label any deviation from "the standards of strength, quality, and purity in the United States Pharmacopoeia and the National Formulary."[117] Drug makers could face criminal prosecution for inaccurate labels. Despite having loopholes that makers of patent medicines could exploit, the law made progress against blatant fraud.

The emphasis of the law on proper labeling of food and drugs was not ideal from Wiley's point of view. The approach assumed that, with adequate information, consumers could protect themselves against the dangers of adulterated food and mislabeled drugs.[118] The law did not include general and easily enforceable standards for adulteration. Instead, if the Bureau of Chemistry should discover adulteration or misbranding of a food or drug, the offender would be informed and allowed to present a case for the adulteration at a hearing. If the evidence indicated violation of the law, the appropriate United States district attorney would be informed to prosecute the offender.[119] The tedious process required defining standards for each case.[120] This limitation did not dampen Wiley's enthusiasm for finally having a law,[121] but it would create problems of enforcement down the road.

Wiley rightly claimed a good part of the credit for passage of the Pure Food and Drug Act. He wrote that in testimony before

Congress, "I took up the arguments that had been advanced by the opponents of the bill and nailed them one by one, figuratively, to the committee table. I summarized the case I had made against adulterants and impurities through the long years of service and the intricate and extended experiments in the Bureau of Chemistry."[122] With the act, he could declare victory in a battle that lasted nearly a quarter of a century. Others agreed, noting that Wiley drafted most of the law as well as giving testimony, speaking in behalf of pure food, and working with organizations to generate widespread support for the legislation.[123] No wonder that many called the legislation the Wiley Act.

President Roosevelt likewise received much credit. The legislation remains one of the major accomplishments of his administration, and his support, however late it came, proved critical for passage of the bill. But tensions persisted in the partnership of Roosevelt and Wiley. They had much in common as pro-business, progressive Republicans who favored more federal regulation of the market. They might have taken joint pride in collaborating on the passage of a food safety law. However, past antagonism and the desire of each to take full credit for the law hindered cooperation. When Roosevelt signed the Meat Inspection Act and the Pure Food and Drug Act in 1906 in a single ceremony, he neglected to mention Wiley. Later he would take credit for getting the bill through Congress, saying that Wiley and his allies were too impractical to overcome the political resistance.[124] Conversely, Wiley viewed Roosevelt as a latecomer to the campaign who received undue credit for passage of the law.[125]

Enforcement

As the chief administrator of the new law, Wiley took the offensive. He organized a staff of inspectors and analysts, mostly young men who shared Wiley's zeal for the crusade.[126] The law was vague enough to give Wiley some freedom in interpreting it, and he willingly used the power to, in his view, protect consumers. "When a member of his staff pointed out that a certain action he proposed was not authorized in the law, Wiley exclaimed: 'But we must read it into the law!'"[127]

Most manufacturers and food sellers adjusted their business to the new law, but there were plenty of exceptions who vigorously fought to block enforcement. Wiley singled out distillers of whiskey, producers of saccharin, and users of sulfur dioxide (to bleach and preserve sugar) as obstructionists. He also said that the makers of patent medicines howled the most about the law and proved to be daunting opponents.[128] As the symbolic leader of the law, Wiley stood out as an inviting target. Opponents tried everything they could, outside of a direct bribe, to get him to ease up on them. Some years later, Wiley wrote that by nature he was not one to quarrel, but he became belligerent when fighting for what he thought was right.[129] If the first claim sounds dubious, the next one rings true.

Despite his efforts, Wiley ultimately failed to implement stringent food and drug safety standards. The real problem came less from the manufactures than from others in government, particularly some in the Department of Agriculture who, in bureaucratic power struggles common in Washington, sought to counteract what they viewed as Wiley's excessive and headstrong actions. Manufacturers exploited the division by bringing complaints about Wiley directly to Agriculture Secretary Wilson. In moving to weaken Wiley's authority, Wilson appointed a Board of Food and Drug Inspection that would have enforcement powers and a Referee Board of Consulting Scientific Experts to make scientific judgments.[130] Despite the accomplished officials and distinguished scientists on the two boards, Wiley saw the changes as a power grab to overturn his work and prevent enforcement of the new law. "I soon found it impossible to bring any cases against certain classes of offenders, particularly the rectifiers and manufacturers of so-called patent medicines containing alcohol as the chief ingredient."[131]

President Roosevelt joined the bureaucratic infighting when makers of benzoate of soda, saccharin, and alum visited the White House. They expressed their concern about the damage from Wiley's vigorous enforcement of the law. When Wiley and Wilson were summoned to the White House to meet with representatives of the manufacturers, Roosevelt accepted Wiley's strongly held view that benzoate of soda was harmful to health. Then Roosevelt asked about saccharin, which the manufacturers used instead of sugar in many products. Wiley told the president it was harmful. In Wiley's telling, "When I said this, President Roosevelt turned upon me, purple with anger, and with clenched fists, hissing through his teeth, said: 'You say saccharin is injurious to health? Why, Doctor Rixey gives it to me every day. Anybody who says saccharin is injurious to health is an idiot.' Our victory was turned into ignominious defeat."[132] Roosevelt upheld Wilson's creation of the Referee Board to advise the Agriculture Department on the safety of food additives.

Both Wilson and Roosevelt worried that Wiley was appropriating too much power, but his national support prevented a direct attack.[133] Instead, the Board of Food and Drug Inspection adopted a less vigorous enforcement strategy that Wiley thought was wholly inadequate. The board moved slowly in developing a strong legal case before threatening action against food manufacturers, while Wiley wanted quick action to protect the consumer by getting as many cases as possible before the court.[134]

More troubles were to come for Wiley. Enemies in the Department of Agriculture charged him with misuse of public funds and called for him to resign. The charges revealed how intensely Wilson and others in the department felt about ousting him.[135] Wiley fought back by accusing his opponents of blocking enforcement of the new law at the behest of commercial interests. When the charges were published in the *New York Times*, the story had the headline "Firing Pure Food Champion—Wiley Refuses to Resign.[136] The public largely took Wiley's side. President William Taft, who replaced Roosevelt in 1909, was inundated with resolutions and letters in support for Wiley, including many from Taft's Republican Party supporters.[137] The president ultimately exonerated Wiley in 1911, concluding that there was no evidence of a conspiracy to defraud the government.[138] Wiley kept his job but could see that his effectiveness had been damaged, and he thought seriously about leaving.

In hindsight, conflict over the law was inevitable. The scientific issues were too complex and the interested parties too varied to lay out precise enforcement details.[139] Not surprisingly, a battle over compliance followed, and Wiley made enemies with his vigorous enforcement.[140] Others might have accepted gaps in enforcement as an unavoidable part of compromise, but Wiley's crusading nature made that difficult. He would become increasingly embittered over the failure to reach his goals.

Pasteurization

The Pure Food and Drug Act made it illegal to add harmful chemicals such as formaldehyde to milk. But the law applied to interstate commerce and mostly to manufactured products. Because milk was sold locally and depended on city and state laws, federal enforcement efforts gave it less attention than other products. Cities and states would have to pass their own laws protecting the purity and quality of milk, meaning that comprehensive change would come slowly.

The Bureau of Chemistry was not well equipped to deal with the problem that, even without harmful chemical additives, milk was prone to carry deadly diseases. By the late 1800s, experts knew much about the source of milk-borne diseases from the research of Pasteur and Koch on bacteria. They knew that milk could spread scarlet fever, diphtheria, typhoid, and tuberculosis and that fermented milk products such as cheese and yogurt did not spread the diseases.[141] They also knew that pasteurization of milk—heating it to just below boiling for twenty minutes—would kill bacteria and, with proper refrigeration, make it considerably safer to drink.[142]

That knowledge led to a debate rather than consensus on how to best protect milk quality. The two sides were both well meaning. If proponents of the Pure Food and Drug Act could be depicted as devoted to public well-being and opponents as greedy businessmen, the lines in the debate over milk were less clearly drawn. Both sides favored public safety but differed over the best means to reach that goal. The outcome shaped the future of food safety, though it would not end the disagreement.

On one side were advocates of pasteurization, mostly businessmen and philanthropists. They said that universal pasteurization made sense as the most practical and reliable way to protect milk. Producers could pasteurize their milk relatively cheaply and efficiently. On the other side were advocates of certification, mostly physicians.[143] They said that pasteurization ruined the taste and degraded the nutrients of raw milk. A healthier and more nutritious approach would be to create a process to certify milk as safe. To obtain certification, dairies would undergo inspection. Buyers would have assurance that certified raw milk was produced under conditions that met quality and safety standards.

In the New York and New Jersey area, a physician named Henry Coit led the certification movement. In searching for safe milk for his newborn child, who could not be breastfed, Coit found the conditions of the dairies he visited to be appalling.[144] With other physicians, he formed a Medical Milk Commission in 1893, which contracted with local dairies to produce milk meeting commission requirements. The group had some success in promoting certification of raw milk. In 1906, the American Association of Medical Milk Commissions was established, and in 1909 New Jersey passed a law protecting the professional activities of milk commissions in the state.[145]

The leader of the pasteurization movement was Nathan Straus, who co-owned Macy's department store. He devoted decades of his life as a philanthropist to championing pasteurization of milk.[146] He believed that pasteurization provided a relatively straightforward fix to the problem compared with bringing thousands of dairies up to the certification requirements. To help poor, working families living in the tenements of New York City, he organized milk depots to distribute low-priced pasteurized milk. Straus would sell the milk below cost, covering the difference from his own funds.[147]

Pasteurization advocates eventually won the debate. In 1908, the surgeon general documented that most childhood deaths came from impure milk and concluded that pasteurization was the best way to address the problem.[148] By 1914, about 88 percent of the milk supply in New York City was pasteurized.[149] In 1924, the Public Health Service published a document that became the Grade A Pasteurized Milk Ordinance, which laid out uniform sanitation standards for the interstate shipment of Grade A milk. The pasteurization ordinance served as the basis for milk safety laws as states and cities across the country adopted the standards.[150] Many states outlawed raw milk altogether; others allowed purchase only at the farms where it was produced; and only a few allowed purchases at the store.[151]

Debate continues over the value of pasteurized milk, and many laud the health-promoting benefits of raw milk. But the widespread use of pasteurization did much to protect the public from the risks of disease, much as the Pure Food and Drug Act protected the public from harmful food additives. As Kurlansky argues, "pasteurization was a public health decision, not a medical one."[152] Certification of raw milk was difficult and expensive, while pasteurization was cheaper, easier to confirm, and more appropriate as a broad public health practice.

Life after the USDA

For most of his life in Washington, DC, Wiley lived simply. He rented a bedroom in the home of a family in the city. As a bachelor, he enjoyed spending time with the family where he lived and socializing in clubs in the city.[153] It was not until 1898, at age fifty-four, that he became serious about marriage. He ran into a young woman, Anna Campbell Kelton, working at the library of the Department of Agriculture. Struck on first sight by her beauty and bearing, he told his companion that he would marry the woman.[154] Kelton was educated, with a degree from Columbian College of George Washington University, and an advocate of women's rights—traits that Wiley found attractive. He managed to have her moved into the job of being his private secretary.[155]

Although Wiley made his romantic interest clear, Kelton remained ambivalent.[156] She did not accept Wiley's proposal for marriage in 1900, telling him that she worried about maintaining her independence. Wiley asked her to keep an open mind, but during a trip he took to France, she left the Department of Agriculture for a job at the Library of Congress. Wiley bided his time, saying, "I saw her only occasionally for the next ten years but during all that time her picture was safely hidden in the back of my watch, and my original determination was unchanged."[157]

In 1910, they again met by chance, this time on a streetcar. Wiley still carried her picture with him.[158] The meeting revived the relationship. When Wiley confessed his continued love, Anna Kelton, who had remained single, was receptive. They married in 1911, when Wiley was sixty-seven and Kelton thirty-three, and would have two sons, Harvey Jr. and John. By all accounts, the marriage worked well. As much as the new Mrs. Wiley supported her husband's crusade for improved food safety, Wiley supported his wife in the crusade for women's right to vote. When Anna Wiley was arrested in 1917 for joining a suffragette protest outside the White House, Wiley expressed pride in her actions.[159] She would outlive her husband by thirty-four years, continuing to act in behalf of progressive causes.[160]

Wiley's marriage was a welcome source of joy in the face of the continuing troubles he encountered in trying to enforce the Pure Food and Drug Act. Still frustrated by the ability of opponents of the law to get the decisions of the Chemistry Bureau overruled, Wiley decided to resign. Staying seemed futile—he could continue the battle more effectively elsewhere.

He wrote a letter of resignation in March 1912 but wanted to submit the letter personally to Secretary Wilson. In a meeting with Wilson, Wiley said he would stay if his enemies in the department were removed.[161] Wilson refused the demand, gladly accepting the resignation. Co-workers were saddened to hear the news, many crowding into his office to wish him well. Some outside the government were outraged, seeing the resignation as a victory for the forces obstructing enforcement of the Pure Food and Drug Act.[162] Mostly, though, the press and the public used the occasion to laud his accomplishments.[163]

Leaving the government ended his long-standing ties to the Republican Party. His anger led him to vote for the first time for a Democratic candidate, Woodrow Wilson, in the 1912 election. Wiley accused Roosevelt of subverting the Pure Food and Drug Act by favoring a few mercenary manufacturers over consumers. In harsh words, he said that the Republican Party had become subjugated by the dollar and big business.[164]

The pull of a new job was likely as important as the frustration of his current job in his decision to leave the government. *Good*

Housekeeping, a magazine that had for some time lent support to the food safety campaign, offered him a position. The offer to direct a new department of food, health, and sanitation doubled his salary and came with some attractive perks. He would have a new lab for food analysis, a regular column in the magazine, and the opportunity to book paid speaking engagements.[165] He would stay at the job for eighteen years, all the while continuing to educate the public about the dangers of adulterated food and dishonest claims about food quality. Most famously, he developed the Good Housekeeping Seal of Approval for products that, based on tests in the magazine's lab, met standards for quality and safety. The seal remains in use today.[166]

Later in life, Wiley published two retrospectives. In one book published in 1929, *The History of a Crime against the Food Law*, he angrily recounted, sometimes in overwhelming detail, the failures of the law and the efforts of opponents to get around its provisions. He published a more upbeat book in 1930, *An Autobiography*, which recounted his life. The autobiography described his early life with nostalgia and showed restraint in reviewing the battles with his enemies. It included a warm and loving acknowledgment to his wife and support for her progressive views.[167]

Wiley died of heart disease in 1930, soon after publishing his autobiography. He lived to age eighty-six, still active to the end. His tombstone in Arlington National Cemetery reads "Father of the Pure Food Law."[168] In 1956, the fiftieth anniversary of the Pure Food and Drug Act, Wiley was honored by a postage stamp with his likeness.[169] More important, his legacy continues today with the activities of the Food and Drug Administration.

The Continuing Food Fight

The Pure Food and Drug Act laid the foundation for the creation of the US Food and Drug Administration. However flawed the legislation was in the details, it represented a momentous shift in policy. It gave the federal government responsibility for the safety of food and the health of the public. Of the progressive accomplishments of Teddy Roosevelt's administration, this one may have had the longest-lasting impact. Wiley became embittered over his failure to enforce the law as he thought was warranted, but in fact the impact of his achievements would be demonstrated in the decades to come.[170]

Enforcement of food safety today traces back to the original Bureau of Chemistry run by Wiley.[171] After reorganization and name changes, the bureau became the US Food and Drug Administration (FDA) in 1930. By that time, the Pure Food and Drug Act had become obsolete, and the FDA recommended in 1933 that it be overhauled. After five years of legislative maneuvering, Congress passed the Federal Food, Drug, and Cosmetic Act in 1938. The law included new regulations for food additives and gave the FDA new powers to enforce the regulations. In 1940, the FDA was transferred to the Federal Security Agency, which became the Department of Health, Education, and Welfare and later the Department of Health and Human Services.

Today, the mission of the FDA is to promote public health by protecting the nation from unsafe foods, drugs, medical devices, and cosmetics. More recently, it took responsibility for regulating the manufacturing, marketing, and distribution of tobacco products.[172] Its leaders view the FDA as a public health agency that relies on the "use of data to identify the riskiest parts of an enormous and complex system" of food supply and distribution.[173] Wiley's Bureau of Chemistry no doubt would endorse these goals.

Since the Pure Food and Drug Act and the Federal Food, Drug, and Cosmetic Act, Congress has passed increasingly stringent regulations for protecting the public from unsafe food.[174] The Food Additives Amendment in 1958 included a clause prohibiting food additives shown to cause cancer in humans or animals.

In 1990, Congress passed the Nutrition Labeling and Education Act that required labeling of packaged food and adherence to federal guidelines in making health claims. In 1996, the Food Quality Protection Act mandated a health-based standard for use of pesticides in food. In 2004, the Food Allergy Labeling and Consumer Protection Act required special labels for foods containing major allergens. The 2009 Food Safety Enhancement Act and the 2011 Food Safety Modernization Act gave the FDA additional powers.

The FDA has been a center of controversy over the enforcement of the new laws, much as the Bureau of Chemistry and Harvey Wiley had been the center of controversy over enforcement of the Pure Food and Drug Act. Problems of food safety are much less severe than in Wiley's time, but battles continue over a multitude of issues relating to cancer-causing food additives, the definition of organic and natural foods, risks and benefits of raw milk, the safety of genetically engineered and irradiated foods, threats of food poisoning from *Salmonella* and *E. coli*, recommended amounts of carbohydrates and fats, the benefits of vegetarian and vegan diets, and the presence of growth hormones in meat, harmful metals in fish, and pesticides in fruits and vegetables.

Despite continuing debates and problems, indisputable progress in food safety has occurred. The Centers for Disease Control and Prevention list improvements in safer and healthier food as one of the ten great public health achievements of the twentieth century.[175] Foods rarely transmit dangerous pathogens, production techniques do more to keep foods fresh and nutritious, and additives are limited to those that are generally recognized as safe. Although hard to quantify, improved nutrition has contributed to the extensions of longevity enjoyed in the past century. The progress is a tribute to the progressive chemist who led the fight for food safety more than one hundred years ago.

4.

The Social Activist
Lillian Wald and Public Health Nursing

It was only a chance visit, but after it occurred, neither nursing nor public health would be the same. At the time, the visit didn't seem special to the nurse, Lillian Wald, or the patient, a Mrs. Lipisky. In 1893, Wald had been teaching a class in New York City to immigrant women.[1] On March 6, after a lesson on bed-making, the daughter of one of the students showed up and asked Wald to visit her mother. It appeared that her mother had recently given birth and was doing poorly. Wald agreed to visit. She had little firsthand experience with the lives of immigrants in the city but followed the girl to one of the tenement buildings on the Lower East Side—a neighborhood filled with poor, mostly Jewish immigrants.

Although Wald felt drawn to helping the needy, her nursing experience had been limited to work in hospitals and an orphanage. She had seen little of the real world of poverty. Raised in a prosperous German-Jewish family in Rochester, New York, she had come to New York City only a few years earlier. She had treated and taught poor patients but had not seen poverty up close.

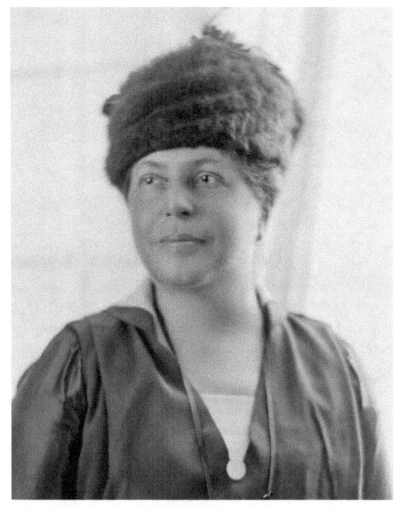

Lillian Wald. *Source*: Wikimedia Commons, from the US Library of Congress, Prints and Photographs Division, Harris and Ewing Collection.

The visit to the home, which was located on Ludlow Street in the Lower East Side, changed that.

The daughter led her over broken roadways and by dirty mattresses and heaps of refuse lying between tall buildings. The streets were filled in all directions with crowds and odors. Wald walked past foul-smelling fish-stands, uncovered garbage cans, and unregulated markets. Once in the building, she walked up slimy tenement steps covered with dirt and mud. She found a family of seven sharing two rooms. The father was disabled and could earn money only by selling cheap products on street corners to sympathetic passersby. The mother "lay on a wretched, unclean bed, soiled with a hemorrhage two days old."[2] Wald cleaned and comforted the woman, earning the family's gratitude.

Wald was shocked by the conditions she saw, although the fault did not lie with the family. They were "neither criminal nor vicious."[3] Rather than being upset by the filthy living conditions themselves, she felt guilty for being part of a society that permitted such conditions to exist. She would write some years later, "All the maladjustments of our social and economic relations seemed epitomized in this brief journey and what was found at the end of it."[4] Naively, she believed at the time that if more people knew about these conditions, they would be sure to end them. She rejoiced in thinking that, as a nurse, she could help with such a project.

The revelation immediately changed the course of her life. She decided to desert the laboratory and academic studies, leave the comfortable student quarters, and devote herself to helping those living in wretched circumstances. Within a day, she had a plan, one she shared with a close colleague, Mary Brewster. "We were to live in the neighborhood as nurses, identify ourselves with it socially, and, in brief, contribute to it our citizenship."[5] She would follow that plan for the rest of her life, but more important, it would enjoy such success as to originate a new form of nursing and a new approach to public health.

Wald would become a model for other young women. Educated, progressive, and independent, they were searching for meaning in their lives. As early feminists, the women wanted to step outside the norms of respectable female behavior to bring about social reform. They retained "a place within the genteel world" of the middle class while gaining political power to bring about the changes they desired.[6]

Nurses had a well-deserved reputation of caring for others in need. But Wald developed something new, what she called public health nursing. She and others like her brought their work from hospitals and private households of the rich to the homes and neighborhoods of the poor, to those most in need of help. Public health nurses did more than treat disease; they sought to instill healthy living habits among their patients and organize the resources of the community to improve the well-being of all the residents. They brought an integrated approach to public health.[7]

The model proved successful. It gained such prominence that Wald and others founded the National Organization for Public Health Nursing in 1912. Public health nursing continues today as a way of complementing the bedside treatment of individual patients with a focus on the environment in which people live. It is defined as "the practice of promoting and protecting the health of populations using knowledge from nursing, social, and public health sciences."[8] It emphasizes prevention, community health, policy advocacy, and social justice.

Much as in Wald's time, public health nursing today is especially concerned with population health disparities. Inequalities in health have been present for centuries, but it is deeply distressing that they remain so sizable after two centuries of progress in extending life and expanding wealth. The nature of the inequality has changed from vulnerability to infectious diseases to vulnerability to chronic diseases. Despite such change, inequalities in health have stubbornly endured. Wald's goal to eradicate these disparities remains an aim of public health nursing, and recent decades have seen calls to reinvigorate Wald's vision.[9]

The Troubling Persistence of Health Inequality

Rudolf Virchow, a German physician who lived from 1821 to 1902, is best known as the father of modern pathology. A polymath, he published more than two thousand scientific writings on pathology, biology, anthropology, prehistory, politics, and—particularly important—what he called "social medicine." In 1848, he was asked to investigate a typhus outbreak in Upper Silesia, an area of modern-day Poland but part of Prussia at the time. Virchow was quite blunt in his assessment: "For there can now no longer be any doubt that such an epidemic dissemination of typhus had only been possible under the wretched conditions of life that poverty and lack of culture had created in Upper Silesia. If these conditions were removed, I am sure that epidemic typhus would not recur."[10] The solution to the epidemic thus came from education, liberty, and prosperity rather than from patient treatment, drugs, or regulation of food, housing, and clothing. Virchow enunciated in brief form what could be seen as the foundation of social medicine: "Medicine is a social science and politics is nothing more than medicine on a large scale."[11] The statement has been called "public health's biggest idea."[12]

The vulnerability of people living in poverty to infectious disease has been obvious throughout history. Edwin Chadwick knew that unsanitary living conditions were most common in poor areas, and John Snow recognized that drinking water was most often infected in low-lying areas of cities where poor people lived. Many expressed concern over the high rates of disease in these neighborhoods. Even the well-off worried that slum-dwellers could spread disease to their more affluent neighborhoods. However, both Chadwick and Snow sought technical fixes to the problem by piping out human waste and piping in clean water. Neither addressed the underlying conditions of poverty and inequality.[13]

Virchow called for a different approach. In Upper Silesia, famine had occurred among peasants in previous years as a result of bad weather and poor harvests. Subjugated by the local aristocracy, the peasants had no options other than to starve. Their physical weakness was the proximate cause of the typhus outbreak, but the poverty and social inequality they lived under was the real cause. Much as illness in an individual indicates a disturbance in the body, outbreaks of disease in populations are "indications of large disturbances of collective life."[14] Social inequality was one such major disturbance, one responsible for the typhus epidemic. Ending future epidemics would require reshaping social and economic institutions.

Socioeconomic Status and Health

Insights about the importance of inequality apply more widely than to infectious disease epidemics alone. In most places and times, people and groups of higher socioeconomic status suffer less from disease, live longer, and enjoy a greater sense of healthy well-being than people and groups of lower socioeconomic status. One might expect that as societies grow richer and citizens live longer, the relationship between status and health would disappear. In fact, it has persisted. When diseases such as typhus and tuberculosis, which primarily affected poor people, were eradicated, socioeconomic differences emerged for other illnesses such as heart disease and cancer. The resources available to high socioeconomic groups—money, education, power, social connections—give them wide-ranging health advantages in nearly all types of societies.[15]

Virchow's ideas are reflected in modern public health in the call for treatment of upstream causes of ill health such as poverty and social inequality along with downstream causes related to individual pathology. The metaphor comes from a well-known story. Standing downstream, a physician sees someone who is about to drown being carried down a swift river, dives in to rescue and treat the person, and continues to do the same thing as more and more people float down the river. A little investigation shows that people are being pushed into the river upstream. Stopping the problem upstream would prevent the problems downstream.

The importance of upstream effects on health is demonstrated by trends in health inequality over the past two centuries. A review by economist Dora Costa divides long-term trends in health in the United States into four periods.[16] The first, from the preindustrial period of the 1700s to the early 1800s, had relatively good health and little inequality. Food was widely available, cities were uncrowded, and epidemics were limited to small areas. The second period, from the 1830s to the 1880s, included the Civil War as well as the growth of industrial work, densely packed cities, and poverty. Although a higher standard of living benefited many, disease epidemics spread quickly through cities, especially among poor residents. Rising inequality in health resulted. The third phase, from the 1880s through the early 1900s, saw the implementation of new health technologies, principally improved sanitation and clean drinking water (which had been developed in earlier decades in London). Scientific progress brought new vaccines, greater safety of milk and food, and better standards for personal hygiene. Because these upstream improvements aided vulnerable poor people more than affluent groups, health inequality declined, though by no means disappeared. The fourth period, from the 1930s or 1950s to the present, has seen increasing inequality. During this period, effective new health technologies and therapies came in the form of private goods that individuals needed to purchase through health insurance or private means. Other treatments required lifestyle changes that placed the burden on individual action. Income and education and their correlates contributed substantially to improved health, and inequalities rose.

Over time, then, health inequalities have risen, declined, and risen again rather than moved steadily downward. The evidence suggests that greater public investment in protecting the health of indigent people has done the most to reduce health inequality.[17] Attending to upstream societal causes of poor health would target access to quality employment, housing, food, health care, and protection against poverty and discrimination. Lillian Wald certainly would agree. She favored programs to improve living conditions in poor neighborhoods as well as treating individual health problems.

A Historical Case in Point: The Lower East Side

A concrete example of health inequality during a period of relative improvement comes from the Lower East Side of New York City around the turn of the twentieth century. The district, which occupies less than one square mile in Manhattan along the East River, was built up in the 1840s by prosperous German immigrants. Late in the nineteenth century, Russian and Polish Jews settled in the area. Beginning in 1881, anti-Semitic riots in Russia pushed Jews to emigrate to the United States from their homeland. A third of the millions of Russia's Jews were driven out, and the approximate numbers of Jews in the United States rose to three million from three hundred thousand.[18] Most of the immigrants settled in the Lower East Side. By 1900, Russian and Polish Jews had largely replaced the earlier immigrant groups, not just in numbers but in the social life and culture of the neighborhood.[19]

The Jewish immigrants came from small towns in Russia and Poland with little money and few skills. The garment industry in the Lower East Side provided jobs for many of them, though at low wages and under sweatshop conditions. With few other options, quite a few sold goods on the streets from pushcarts, also an occupation with paltry earnings. Children needed to help out. According to a survey, more children worked than attended school.[20] One Israel Beilin was born in Russia, came to the United States at age five, and grew up on Cherry Street in the Lower East Side. After only a few years of schooling, Israel began to work by selling newspapers as an eight-year-old. As a teenager, he took a job as a singing waiter to support himself. It turned out that he had a knack for composing songs that pleased his customers. Although he later became famous as Irving Berlin, one of America's greatest songwriters, his childhood reflects the difficult times in the Lower East Side.

The lives of Jewish children were dominated by crowded living conditions in the tenements of the Lower East Side and by crowded streets outside the tenements. Families lived in buildings that had been subdivided into small and poorly maintained apartments. Here is how one historian describes the living conditions:

> abominably crowded homes, people reduced to living in cellars, without windows or light, sleeping in hallways, on roofs or fire-escapes, unbearable heat and stench in summer, unendurable cold in the winter, filth, noise, outdoor plumbing, endless hours of labor for every member of the family down to the smallest, spectacles of vice flaunted for the children to see, bags of refuse flung out of tenement windows onto the hats of citizens passing below, pushcarts, curses, quarrels, vermin of all sorts, rats, beetles as big as half-dollars, street fights and gang warfare.[21]

The apartments were poorly ventilated, running water was rare, and the small rooms seldom had enough space for everyone to sleep.

The other inescapable part of life in the Lower East Side was the teeming neighborhood streets, which "were congested, packed

with people, carts, and horse-drawn wagons and strewn with manure, garbage, and raw sewage."[22] Lillian Wald gives a sense of
the street life in describing what she saw when looking out her
window at two o'clock in the morning:

> Some of the push-cart venders still sold their wares. Sitting on the
> curb directly under my window, with her feet in the gutter, was a
> woman, drooping from exhaustion, a baby at her breast. The fire-
> escapes, considered the most desirable sleeping-places, were
> crowded with the youngest and the children were asleep on the
> sidewalks, on the steps of the houses and in the empty push-carts;
> some of the more venturesome men and women with mattress or
> pillow staggered toward the riverfront or the parks.[23]

Young people sometimes found the life of the streets to be exciting and adventure-filled, if also somewhat dangerous. But few
would want to stay if they could escape.

The crowding of families inside poorly ventilated tenements,
the workers sitting side-by-side in sweatshops, and the close contact of neighbors while out on the unsanitary streets made the
inhabitants particularly vulnerable to the spread of diseases. Residents feared but could not avoid the White Plague—tuberculosis—
as well as other infectious diseases. High unemployment and poverty exacerbated health problems. The squalid living conditions of
those living in the Lower East Side created a public scandal. Jacob
Riis, a journalist originally from Denmark but now settled in the
United States, had experienced the hardships of immigration
himself. He published an exposé in 1890, *How the Other Half Lives:
Studies among the Tenements of New York*, that mixed stories, statistics, and photos. The statistics were informative. One tenement
in the area housed thirty-six families, with fifty-eight babies and
thirty-eight children over age five.[24] Two small rooms in another
building managed to hold a couple, their twelve children, and six

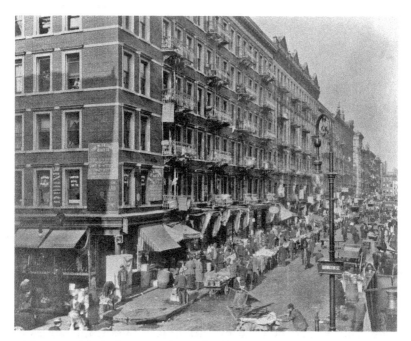

Rivington Street in the Lower East Side of Manhattan, 1909. *Source*:
Wikimedia Commons, from the US Department of Energy.

boarders. More than the text, however, the photos of children
sleeping on an alleyway grate or a man sorting through trash
shocked readers. The photos revealed the distress and despair of
the residents and led to outrage among city leaders, including
Teddy Roosevelt, the police commissioner and future president,
and to some modest reforms by means of the New York Tenement
House Act of 1901.

It was in this neighborhood that Wald would work, officially as
a nurse and unofficially as a social worker, for most of her adult
life. The health care model she developed for the residents of the
Lower East Side laid out a new role for nurses, one that addressed
the social ills causing health problems as well as the health problems themselves.

A New Kind of Nurse

The Professionalization of Nursing

Nursing has a long history, but up to the mid-1800s, it primarily took the form of private care within homes. Nurses had a role similar to family members in caring for a sick person, except that they were paid by those who could afford it.[25] One history of nursing explains, "the paid nurse, whether at home or in hospital, would mostly have given the elementary physical care that a patient in other circumstances might have received from an amateur family member or personal servant."[26] Not needing much technical knowledge, nurses came from the lower classes, much as domestic servants did.

The revolution in nursing care began with Florence Nightingale, who established the first training program for nurses in 1860. Nightingale entered adulthood frustrated by her wealthy, educated, and religious upbringing in Victorian England. She felt that the roles available to women at the time were wholly unsuitable for someone with ambition and talent. She decried "the imprisonment of women's minds with trivial pursuits, stating that women needed meaningful employment or vocations, similar to men."[27] Her strong Christian beliefs directed her toward helping those in need, but that goal was blocked by the Victorian ethos for upper-class women to devote their lives to children, husbands, and household tasks. The extent of her unhappiness is vividly apparent in a note in her diary in 1852: "Why, oh my God, can I not be satisfied with the life that satisfies so many people? I am told that the conversation of all these clever men ought to be enough for me. Why am I so starving, desperate and diseased on it. . . . My God, what am I to do?"[28] Nursing offered a way out of the stultifying life she expected. It was an occupation open to women that could fulfill her desires to help those in need.

Nightingale's mother had forbidden her to become a nurse, which upper-class families not inaccurately viewed as little different from a domestic servant. But Nightingale stubbornly followed her ambition. She rejected one suitor after a long courtship and vowed at age thirty to maintain a life of chastity. With an annuity from her father for support, and a good deal of freedom in her life, she managed to educate herself in nursing. Her first real job, at age thirty-three, was as the superintendent of the Institute for the Care of Sick Gentlewomen in London. While serving there in 1854, Nightingale helped respond to the cholera epidemic and worked briefly with John Snow.[29]

That same year, she found a greater calling for her services. England had been allied with France and Turkey against Russia in the Crimean War of 1853 to 1856. Stories about the terrible conditions of wounded English soldiers shocked the public in England. Invited to help by the minister of war, a close friend, Nightingale jumped at the chance to make a difference in the world. She led a team of thirty-eight women to the military hospital located on the Asian side of Istanbul.[30] She found an overworked staff and soldiers who died more often from the spread of infections and the lack of hygiene, good food, and medicine than from their wounds. A champion of sanitary control, "She and her nurses meticulously swept, scrubbed, laundered clothes, made bandages from clean cloth, and managed safe food supplies."[31] Proving to be skilled at organizing her staff and devising an orderly system of care, Nightingale instituted changes that, according to many reports, greatly reduced the death rate.[32]

Publicity about her accomplishments led to national celebrity. Called a heroine in newspaper articles, she was depicted as moving through the hospital during nightly rounds to give the soldiers comfort and hope. A Henry Wadsworth Longfellow poem in 1857 refers to the "a lady with a lamp" passing "through the glimmering gloom."[33] By the late 1850s, Nightingale had become perhaps the most famous woman in England, outside of Queen Victoria. Modern biographers suggest that her accomplishments were exaggerated and that her reputation was based on flawed statistics, but there is no disputing her fame.

Returning to London, she used donations from citizens impressed by her work to establish the first Training School for Nurses at St. Thomas Hospital. Based on her experiences in the Crimean War, Nightingale designed the program to emphasize the priority of good sanitation in caring for the sick. The program professionalized nursing by using a standardized curriculum that hospitals could adopt. She was also concerned about the reliance on untrained nurses for home care outside the hospital. Only professionally trained nurses, who had learned the principles of sanitary care in hospitals, could provide suitable care to those sick at home. An innovative statistician and epidemiologist as well as a nurse, Nightingale collected data demonstrating that most home nurses were untrained.[34] Owing to Nightingale's efforts, nursing steadily became a more respectable profession than when she first entered the field.

To provide high-quality nursing outside the hospital, Nightingale set up a system of district nursing. After receiving proper training in modern principles of care, nurses would go to the homes of patients in their district but do more than treat the sickness. Nightingale believed that the district nurse should be a health missioner who taught health as well as delivered treatment.[35] Learning the practices of hygiene, principles of sanitation, and importance of fresh air and good diet would help patients recover and protect themselves from illness. The approach added health education and social work to the role of sick care. She believed, naively no doubt, that proper nursing of the sick in their own homes plus a good dose of primary prevention would eventually lead to the abolition of hospitals.[36]

Nightingale noted the differences between hospital and home nursing. Nursing in hospitals demanded discipline, subordination, and following orders. Nursing in homes allowed for more independence and reliance on personal qualities and skills; it was suited for women from higher social classes who had the educational background to complete more rigorous training and operate with a good deal of autonomy.[37] Indeed, the work of the nurse in the field came closer to that of the physician. As Nightingale wrote, "a district nurse must be even a better trained nurse than a hospital nurse, because she has so much less help at hand. There must be nothing of the amateur about her. She has not the doctor always at hand."[38]

In the United States, three nursing schools that followed the formal training inspired by Florence Nightingale opened in New York, Boston, and New Haven, Connecticut, in 1873.[39] The first nursing graduate, Linda Richards, received training at the New England Hospital for Women and Children in Boston and went to London to work with Nightingale. The number of nursing schools expanded quickly. By 1890, there were thirty-five schools with 1,552 nursing students.[40]

Desire for Adventure

Although born forty-seven years later than Florence Nightingale, Wald shared many of the same traits and views. Both were most obviously devoted to nursing and to expanding and improving the profession. Both were skilled executives able to organize and supervise a large staff. Both were feminists who rejected the traditional role of wife and mother and worked for women's rights. Both came from privileged backgrounds but used their advantages to help others. And both were natural, even charismatic, leaders who were devoted to social reform and human rights. Each helped to reshape and advance nursing, although in somewhat different ways.

Wald came of age as part of a progressive generation in America that pioneered new social roles for women.[41] Not having access to the same jobs as men, women of this generation devised new occupations that took advantage of their education and met their needs for meaningful work outside the home. Their accomplishments changed public policy and social institutions. Much as Harvey Wiley brought progressive values to food safety, Wald brought these values to nursing.

Given that she would rebel against the roles for women of her mother's generation, it may be surprising that Wald had a happy childhood. She was close to her parents, who tended to spoil and indulge her, and she spoke lovingly about the warmth and comfort of her family.[42] Born in 1867 to German-Jewish parents, Max and Minnie, Wald grew up in affluence in Cincinnati, Ohio, and then from ages eleven to twenty-two in Rochester, New York. Her father owned a successful optical company. Thoroughly assimilated, the parents had little or no contact with immigrants, poor people, or traditional Judaism. In a pleasant, middle-class home, Wald grew up as a "strong, happy, curious child."[43] Enjoying life in a close-knit family as she did, Wald might have wanted to carry on the same happy life of her childhood and youth by marrying, having children, and raising a family—the life her older sister chose.

What made Wald different was an overpowering desire for adventure, for something new and exciting. She excelled in the private Day School for Young Ladies that she attended and, in searching for a new challenge, applied to Vassar College at age sixteen. Turned down as too young, she then occupied herself with music and French lessons, all the while looking for the opportunity to do something more, to break away from what others expected of her. She was popular, attractive, and received a lot of attention.[44] While Wald was never prone to introspection or self-analysis, it seems clear that the world in which she was raised did not satisfy her ambition.[45]

One event gave her a vision of what she could achieve. During the birth of her older sister's child, which took place in the family home, a nurse came to help. Seeing the nurse in action, Wald experienced "an irresistible impulse" to become a nurse.[46] She saw the "opening of a window on the new world," something suitable for women experiencing a restless discontent with traditional roles.[47] She could help people, have a challenging career, and work in an occupation that welcomed women. Her parents disliked the idea of a nursing career. Like Nightingale's parents, they viewed the work as dangerous and degrading for someone from her station.[48] Only reluctantly did her father and mother come to accept her goal.

In 1889, at age twenty-two, Wald left Rochester for a career in nursing. Hoping to receive training at the New York Hospital in Manhattan, she wrote to the superintendent. Her letter said that a life devoted to "society, study, and house keeping duties" no longer satisfied her. She felt "the need of serious, definite work."[49] Indeed, as part of the new direction she planned for her life, Wald readily gave up the luxuries she enjoyed in Rochester.[50] Happiness would come not from comfortable affluence but from fellowship and close bonds with other women who shared her goals to do something authentic and pioneering.

Wald moved to New York City, entered the nursing training at the hospital, and graduated in 1891. New York Hospital stood out as one of the first in the United States to implement Nightingale's program for nurse training. She referred to graduating as one of her proudest moments.[51] She learned to maintain self-control and stay calm in the face of stress and crisis at the hospital, but she chafed under the rigid discipline and tight supervision faced by its nurses.[52] Not wanting to work as an underling in a hospital or as a private nurse in the homes of the wealthy, she took a job in 1891 at an orphanage, the New York Juvenile Asylum. Her experience there "left her dismayed, forever embittered toward institutional care for children."[53] She loved the children but was appalled by their mistreatment.[54] With the hope for a career with more freedom, she began medical school at Women's Medical College of the New York Infirmary. However, the discrimination against women physicians that she saw discouraged her.[55]

During her time in medical school, Wald began to teach a course on homemaking for immigrant women living in the Lower East Side. The contact with Jewish immigrants fortified her belief in universalism, that immigrants were like everyone else.[56] They needed only time to become comfortable with a new culture. Such was the attitude she brought to the visit with Mrs. Lipisky that changed the direction of her life.

The House on Henry Street

After her experience in the home of Mrs. Lipisky, Wald immediately set out to realize her vision to serve the poorest residents of the Lower East Side of New York City. She and her collaborator, Mary Brewster, sought to create a place in the neighborhood where they could offer community-wide nursing. They knew that about 90 percent of the sick people in cities remained in their homes and needed care.[57] But they wanted to do more than treat the sick. They wanted to become involved with the social life of the neighborhood, to create a sense of community and contribute to nonmedical needs. They wanted to be full members of the locality, to provide neighborly and democratic services. Yet, they knew little about the district or the world outside the hospital.[58]

As a first step in 1893, they rented rooms on the top floor of a building on Jefferson Street in the Lower East Side. The search for accommodations proved frustrating. Both women wanted a bathroom and bathtub—a rarity in the neighborhood.[59] Once they succeeded in their search and started to make their presence known, people came looking for help with their health problems.[60] The facilities turned out to be too small to meet the needs of the community, however.

Fortunately, Wald found a wealthy sponsor and a strong supporter of her goals. Jacob Schiff, a German-Jewish banker who was born in Frankfurt, had come to the United States in 1865. Joining an investment bank on Wall Street, he helped finance the expansion of business during the Gilded Age of the late 1800s. Enormously wealthy, he devoted time and money to charitable support for Jewish causes. Schiff much admired the work that Wald had begun on the Lower East Side. He not only donated to the program but also became a role model and father figure to Wald.[61] He would introduce her to other donors in upper-class society of New York City.

With funds provided by Schiff, Wald bought a house in 1895 at 265 Henry Street, located in the middle of the district. When built in 1827, the house was part of a street populated by middle-class merchants who did business in the nearby South Street Seaport.[62] The houses on the street were stately, constructed with sturdy doors, beautiful details, and impressive woodwork. Over time, as the middle-class residents moved to newer neighborhoods, Henry Street and its environs attracted immigrants. Landlords subdivided the once-fine homes into tenement apartments. The house Schiff bought for Wald had been preserved better than most. Photos show a handsome, three-story, red brick building with many large windows.

The house had room for many nurses but needed remodeling.[63] The ground floor was set up as a public space where Wald and others could treat health problems and hold meetings with the public. The second floor contained a dining room and sitting room for individual meetings. Wald and Brewster took the top floor of the three-story building for their bedrooms so that they could both live and work in the same location. Other nurses also lived in the building, occupying small rooms originally built for servants.

Before anything else, Wald and Brewster wanted to build trust with the neighborhood residents.[64] Toward that end, they complemented nursing care by supplying "small loans, food, job referrals, carfare, [and] emotional support" to those in need, much as social workers would do.[65] Although the women worked most closely with the Jewish residents of the neighborhood, the assistance was nonsectarian in nature—all were welcome.[66] The help came with a special form of patient empowerment.[67] The goal was to guide and encourage the clients and patients rather than simply fix their problems.

The settlement houses that had sprung up around the country in previous decades served as a model for the Henry Street House. Settlement houses, typified by Hull House, founded in Chicago by Jane Addams, aimed to bring the classes together by having well-off and poor people live in close physical proximity. The houses were located in poor areas but inhabited by middle-class settlement workers. They provided services to those in need while developing ties to the neighborhood. The term "settlement" came from the goal of settling in the area. Workers lived among those being served rather than commuting in each day and returning to homes in middle-class neighborhoods.[68] Services thus came from fellow residents of the neighborhood rather than from traditional charities that delivered aid from the outside.

Leadership made up largely of women also distinguished settlement houses. Ellen Snyder-Grenier provides some informative statistics: "Three-fifths of American settlement residents between 1889 and 1914 were female. Ninety percent had been to college, part of the early generation of American college-educated women."[69] The houses offered opportunities to educated and middle-class women that they could not find elsewhere.[70] The meaningful work, the opportunities for leadership, and the connections with other women who shared the same values attracted progressive women. They could not yet vote, but as part of the settlement house movement, they could take action on issues important to them. Wald lauded "the settlement as the most pliable tool for social service that has been developed."[71]

While adopting the settlement house model, Wald reshaped it to match her own plans. She added nursing and health care as primary goals of the house and initially hired a staff of six nurses committed to the same vision of helping those in need.[72] The Henry Street House invited neighbors to visit, but more important, Wald and the staff went out to the homes of the neighborhood residents. They could then treat health problems of patients confined to their homes as well as teach home-based sanitary and hygienic practices. Equally significant, the nurses could become part of the lives of the families they helped. Although committed first to nursing care, the Henry Street House offered many other forms of aid. The approach excited and motivated the nursing staff. They not only shared a residence and living expenses but also a sense of promise and adventure.[73]

Exceptional Organizational and Leadership Skills

Wald appears to have been liked and admired by all who knew her. She had a group of close friends and co-workers plus a wide network of acquaintances throughout the city and country. As a leader, she is described as charismatic, visionary, innovative, inspiring, and passionate.[74] As a person, she is described as attracting people from all walks of life with her laughter, "exuberance, charm, and warmth," and as having "inordinate capacity for loving people of all sorts."[75] In pursuing her goals, particularly in her efforts to attract wealthy donors, she managed to combine friendly persuasion with unbending persistence.[76]

Wald's exceptional organizational and leadership skills, although based on idealistic goals, helped her get things done. Outreach was always central. Early on, she arranged dinners at Henry Street where, sitting at the head of the table, she would talk to the guests about the mission and activities of the house. Invitees came from all walks of life and helped form a bridge across the social classes in the city.[77] Over the decades, she spent more time on administration and funding-raising and less time as a nurse and in contact with neighborhood residents.[78] As a fund-raiser, she attended receptions in the city's opulent mansions, comfortably mixed with city leaders, and spoke to wealthy donors about supporting the Henry Street House. She gave many speeches, joined committees, and founded organizations. She mixed with the poor immigrants who lived in the neighborhood, with the educated and independent nurses who worked with her, and with the politicians and upper-class residents of the city who supported the Henry Street House. Few could co-operate so well with such a diverse coalition of supporters.

Although Wald worked closely with men, her strongest ties were with other women. She believed that women had natural strengths that set them apart from men.[79] Their sense of maternal warmth and generosity was well suited for the healing and helping role. Rigorous training as a nurse and demanding work provided an outlet for nurses to have independent careers while allowing them to use their special aptitudes. In combining independence with caring for the poor and sick, Wald effectively mixed modern and traditional roles.

Her attitudes fostered strong feelings of sisterhood, not only with other nurses but also with women and mothers in the neighborhood. She developed what might be called an "old girl network,"[80] which sought to elevate the status of women. Settlement houses, generally led and staffed by women, served as venues for political action. The women supported women's suffrage, equal opportunity for women, and removal of the barriers women faced in access to schooling, jobs, and politics. Settlement houses also supported a variety of progressive causes related to fair housing, safe working conditions, and regulation of business. Wald fully agreed with these views.

Given her views about essential differences between men and women, Wald never became a militant feminist.[81] "She preferred cooperation and conciliation over militant action."[82] Being pragmatic in her desire to achieve practical goals, she had no desire to alienate her supporters, including wealthy donors, with radical attacks.[83] Her views stayed solidly in the mainstream. She fit best within the liberal Progressive ethos of the time that sought a stronger, more interventionist role of government within the existing democratic framework.[84]

Wald was tall for the time, five feet and seven inches, and attractive. Daniels describes her as "vain about her appearance" and maintaining "an interest in dress and style."[85] She developed long-term, intimate, and very private relationships with women that have led some historians to suggest that Wald had several lesbian relationships.[86] She certainly felt fulfilled by her closeness to other women, having never married or developed deep relationships with men.[87] In any case, Wald's nonstop work left little time to fully commit to an intimate partnership, which some of her closest friends found frustrating.[88]

Public Health Innovations

The Henry Street House grew steadily after its founding. In the short period from 1901 to 1910, starting only six years after its founding, the staff grew from fifteen to fifty-four nurses. The nurses attended to 3,000 patients in 1901, while in 1910 they "made 143,589 home visits and administered 18,934 first aid treatments."[89] The success came in good part from the "impressive if disjointed array of services" provided to the neighborhood.[90] Along with nursing, Wald and her team organized clubs, classes, physical activities for children such as camps and playgrounds, and civic work such as fighting for cleaner streets, better schools, more parks, and improved housing.[91]

Wald brought several long-lasting innovations to public health through the Henry Street House—a visiting nurse system, school nurses, private insurance for home care, and a coordinated, data-based response to epidemics.

Public Health Nursing

A 1908 photo shows a young woman on the rooftop of a tenement building. She is dressed in white, with a full-length skirt, long-sleeved and neck-high blouse, and a wide-brimmed hat. She is also carrying a small black bag. The woman, using a crate as a step-stool, is about to climb over a short wall that separates one rooftop from another. The juxtaposition of a properly dressed woman with her surprising location is unusual. But then, so was the woman. She was a visiting nurse from the Henry Street House traveling from one appointment to another. It turns out that walking across rooftops was the best way to visit patients who typically lived in the cheapest apartments on the top floor of the tenements. The nurses found it quicker and easier to walk across rooftops than to walk up and down stairways all day long.

Such was the daily work of the nurses at the Henry Street House. Delivering proper care required nurses to make home visits. Poor people viewed hospitals as places of last resort, where the sick went to die.[92] Those unable to pay for a physician's visit received no care until it was too late to recover. Then, when little more could be done, patients went to the hospital. Wald saw that nurses

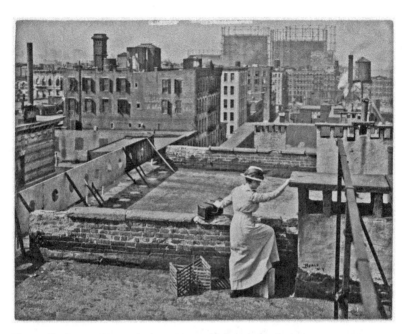

Henry Street nurse crossing tenement rooftops, 1908. *Source*: VNS Health, New York City, and Columbia University Health Sciences Library.

could prevent more serious illness and death with early home treatment and guidance on healthy living—even if it meant clambering across rooftops.

The nursing philosophy of the Henry Street House stressed the delivery of services with compassion and without judgment.[93] Fees were based on the ability to pay, meaning that many paid nothing at all.[94] The aid would be seen not as charity but as part of the relationship between the nurses and the community. The relationships would be personal as well as professional. The nurses became familiar with and respected the culture, language, and customs of those they served. Such reciprocity maintained the dignity and self-respect of the patients.[95]

The distinctive occupation of the Henry Street nurses had several names. "Visiting nurses," "community nurses," and, to borrow from Nightingale, "district nurses" all fit. But Wald wanted a new name that would better define the goals and activities of her staff. The term "public health nurse" described nursing practices that linked care and treatment to community action.[96] In Wald's own words, "The call to the nurse is not only for bedside care of the sick, but to help in seeking out the deep-lying basic causes of illness and misery, that in the future there may be less sickness to nurse and cure."[97] Public health nurses visited homes, lived in the community, served those in need, taught healthful living, and assisted in ways that improved the overall well-being and prevented future health problems.

The nurses faced a demanding workload to meet the public health goals. Karen Buhler-Wilkerson describes their day.[98] At breakfast, the nurses planned their schedule and discussed any special problems they would face. Wald assigned new cases, although leaving the nurses free to manage their patients and schedules. After daily rounds of visiting patients in the morning, the nurses returned for lunch, went out again for afternoon rounds, and then returned to the house later in the day for other activities such as teaching English classes and running a club for teenage girls. The nurses needed diverse skills. "They alleviated distressing symptoms, intervened in emergencies, gave necessary treatments, brought the latest in portable medical technology, provided health education to all ages, and were welcomed visitors," and they contributed "clothes, food, equipment, child care, housekeeping services, and assistance to exhausted family income providers in need of relief from caregiving responsibilities."[99]

In 1907, the *New York Times* published an article describing the day of one Henry Street nurse.[100] The nurse began the morning by climbing across three or four boats to reach a pneumonia patient living in a canal boat and then went to an apartment to bathe a newborn baby and help the recently widowed mother. She next met with an elderly man who had leg problems but really wanted to talk with someone. In two more visits, she helped a disabled woman care for her home and her son and comforted a dying Italian man whose wife and daughter needed to keep sewing garments to support the family. After lunch, the pace was equally hectic: visiting the pneumonia patient on the boat again and arranging for a night nurse to help; bringing flowers and checking on a young girl recuperating from an illness and explaining to the mother how to give the needed medicine; and finding someone to do sewing for the Italian women so they could care for the dying husband and father. No wonder the patients and their families adored the visiting nurses.

The independence of the visiting nurses created one new and potentially serious problem—friction with physicians. Unlike at hospitals, the Henry Street nurses worked without supervision by physicians. They would refer patients to physicians as needed but otherwise acted on their own. Wald and others believed that nursing had reached a level of professionalism to justify their autonomy. But the medical profession generally sought to protect its professional monopoly from the competition of other health providers. To avoid antagonizing the medical profession, Wald tried to keep public clinics separate from private medical practices.[101] At least in public, she said nurses only offered services for problems that were not serious enough for a physician visit or hospitalization and that they did not prescribe medicines.[102]

The adoption of the public health nursing program by other organizations besides the Henry Street House called for a national organization. Wald took the lead. As chair of a 1910 Committee on Visiting Nursing of the American Nurses Association, she led the effort to create the National Organization for Public Health Nursing in 1912.[103] The group had a diverse constituency such as nurses from antituberculosis organizations, rural health agencies, and industrial health units. The name "public health nursing" encompassed the diversity, while the organization gave official

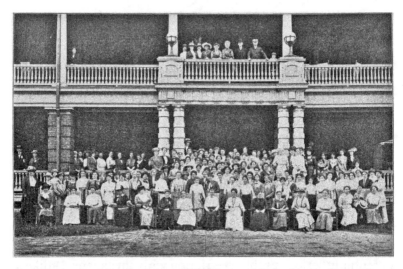

Attendees at the annual meeting of the National Organization for Public Health Nursing, Atlantic City, New Jersey, 1913. *Source*: Wikimedia Commons, from the *Public Health Nurse Quarterly* 5(3) (July 1913).

recognition to the new occupation. With funding from an anonymous donor, the organization hired a full-time director, published the *Visiting Nurse Quarterly*, and worked to establish professional standards and an information clearinghouse. A photograph of attendees at the 1913 meeting of the National Organization for Public Health Nursing in Atlantic City, New Jersey, shows the early interest in the goals Wald set for the association. The organization would continue until 1952, when it helped form the National League for Nursing.[104]

School Nurses

It was hard for Wald not to give special attention to the deprived and vulnerable children in the Lower East Side. She knew that treating and preventing health problems of children would lessen adult problems later. Along with distributing safe milk and food to families, the Henry Street House offered classes for mothers on childcare, hygiene, and first aid.[105] The greater payoff, however, would come from helping children in schools, where they congregated in large numbers.

Laws and regulations in some cities already required medical inspections of schoolchildren to stop the spread of disease.[106] In New York City, physicians checked students for contagious diseases, and those with symptoms were sent home. While partly effective, the inspections were, in Wald's words, "perfunctory and only superficially touched the needs of the children."[107] Many other students who came to school with noncommunicable conditions such as skin disease, eye problems, malnutrition, and physical defects also needed treatment.[108] The thousands of children sent home without treatment because of eye infections ended up playing in the street and likely infecting other children.[109] Even when doctors recommended treatment, parents had trouble understanding the written instructions.[110]

Wald dealt with the problem in 1902 by proposing an experiment to representatives of the New York City Board of Education and Board of Health. A Henry Street nurse, Lina Rogers, would work with four schools for a period of one month to improve children's health and reduce school absenteeism. Wald would pay the salary of Rogers for the first month, and the Board of Health thereafter would take over the costs if the members were pleased with the results.[111] Consistent with the philosophy of public health nurses, Rogers did more than treat health problems. Emphasizing wellness and prevention, she taught students, parents, and teachers about hygiene, nutrition, and exercise. In only one month, she "treated 893 students, made 137 home visits, and helped 25 children who had received no previous medical attention recover and return to school."[112] A few days later, the New York City Board of Education hired Rogers as the nation's first school nurse and then expanded program. The city came to employ nearly four hundred nurses in its schools by 1914, and the practice spread to other localities.[113] By 1911, 102 cities across the country employed school nurses.[114]

Home Care Insurance

Perhaps Wald's most original and, at least initially, far-reaching public health innovation was launching a private insurance program for home care. The program reveals the kind of creative thinking Wald brought to health problems and the wide-ranging contacts she had in the private sector.

The idea came from a 1909 conversation Wald had with Lee Frankel, the recently hired manager of the new Welfare Division of Metropolitan Life Insurance.[115] The two quickly recognized their common interests—Wald to expand visiting nursing and Frankel to provide for the welfare of the company's policyholders. They convinced the company's board of directors that it could cut death-benefit payouts by having nurses visit sick and unhealthy clients. Good prevention would save money. At the start, MetLife agreed to pay the nurses 50 cents per each visit with a sick policyholder.[116] Along with the opportunity to increase profits, the home nursing program would enhance the company's image.

The project began in 1909 as a three-month experiment, and the trial proved successful enough to continue. Statistics showed that insurance sales increased and mortality declined in neighborhoods where the nurses visited. MetLife soon expanded the program throughout New York City and then to other parts of the country.[117] By 1916, with 10.5 million MetLife customers having the home-care policy, the program resembled a national insurance system for home-based care.[118] Wald viewed the evidence that home nursing care saved lives with much satisfaction but also felt some unease. The profit-making demand for efficiency and control over the practitioners conflicted with the benevolent ethos of the visiting nurses.[119] Despite the conflict, the program proceeded steadily, expanding home nursing beyond any conception Wald might have had years earlier.

War and the Spanish Flu Epidemic

By 1917, the year the United States entered World War I, the Henry Street House had become an essential public health resource for the city. It was ready to respond swiftly to the new public health strains placed on the city by the war. Wald no doubt felt frustrated by the new demands. She had long opposed entrance of the United States into the European conflict. She and other suffragettes led the Women's Peace Parade in New York City in 1914. The 1,200 participants marched down Fifth Avenue to express their opposition to joining the war.[120] From 1914 to 1917, Wald served as the chair of the newly formed American Union against Militarism, which would eventually evolve into the American Civil Liberties Union.[121] Yet, when the war came, Wald and the Henry Street House took immediate action. The war effort sent physicians into the armed forces, raised prices for food and heating, and left children and the elderly vulnerable to disease. Working with other service organizations, the Henry Street House did as much as it could to lessen the worsening health of the city's population. It was a busy time for Wald, but the difficulties would intensify.

The war accelerated the spread in 1918-1920 of the so-called Spanish flu, which killed an estimated 25 million people worldwide.[122] The pandemic stands as one of the deadliest in human history. When the flu came to New York City, beginning in the fall of 1918, tens of thousands died. The Henry Street House immediately recognized the seriousness of the crisis. From the very start, it was overwhelmed by families in need of help. Wald wrote that the staff was devoting nearly all nursing care to victims of the flu and pneumonia.[123] Along with providing care, the visiting nurses collected data on the patients they saw.[124] City officials could use the data to effectively target resources where they were most needed.

With her usual energy, Wald took the lead in organizing a co-ordinated response to the epidemic in the city. Appointed as chair of the Nurses Emergency Council, she joined forces with both public and private agencies to mobilize volunteers.[125] Filling key support roles, the volunteers transported nurses, moved supplies, and delivered food. The council sponsored a publicity campaign that included an advertisement in the Sunday papers with the headline, "A Stern Task for Stern Women." It stated, "There is nothing in the epidemic of Spanish influenza to inspire panic. There is everything to inspire coolness and courage and sacrifice on the part of American women. A stern task confronts our women—not only trained women, but untrained women." The appeal ends with a question: "Will you enroll for service now?"[126]

The council instructed nurses on how to protect themselves while caring for the sick and how to help families prevent the disease from spreading to others.[127] The instructions included a plan for establishing after-care stations in small districts and appointing a trained nurse or dietician to take charge of patient after-care in each spot. The stations would recommend a diet for those who could afford their own food and prepare suitable food for those who could not. When needed, the stations would supply milk and eggs. Those in charge of the stations would check for warning symptoms of disease while dispensing food. They might even arrange an outing to the park or country to help patients recover.

Serving All Those in Need

Helping the vulnerable with home-based care and adding a good dose of guidance on hygiene, nutrition, and disease prevention made up one part of the public health mission of Wald and the Henry Street House. The other part related to the broader societal problems that led to health inequalities. This component of the public health mission required social activism. Visiting nurses and home care certainly helped neighborhoods and communities thrive. They brought physical relief and personal comfort to the sick and suffering. But Wald saw the value of more extensive changes in the organization of social and economic life in the city and country. She would have less success changing society than in improving the health of community residents. Social activism nonetheless remained an essential part of her approach to public health.

Children

From the start, Wald wanted to help the children overflowing from the confined spaces of the tenements into the lively, crowded, and in some ways unsafe streets of the Lower East Side. An immediate step was to build a playground in the back yard of the Henry Street House and its environs where children could play safely and get help as needed from the Henry Street House staff.[128] The simple action quickly attracted children from the neighborhood. The space could handle only a tiny portion of the thousands of children roaming the streets, however. Wald also used her contacts and influence to prod the city to do more. She collaborated with city officials to build public playgrounds. The first city-built playground in Seward Park was located just a few blocks from the Henry Street House.[129] When it opened in 1903, twenty thousand children mobbed the gates and rushed in.[130]

In the schools, the nursing program that Wald and Lina Rogers developed did more than improve the health of the children. For one thing, it reduced absenteeism. Past efforts to contain contagious diseases by sending children home often ended up depopulating the schools.[131] Children learned little at home and placed a strain on working parents. After a school nurse helped one student with a skin disease, the mother wrote, "We are very much obliged to you for . . . not sending Sadie home. I am busy working in the store from early morning to late in the night. I will put this salve on her head every night till it is cured."[132] But sick and healthy students alike needed something more—nutritious food. A hungry student, and there were many in poor neighborhoods, was a poor student. In 1908, Wald pushed for free school lunches that would avoid stigmatizing children who needed them.[133]

Outside of school, the neighborhood children could find quiet and restful study rooms plus coaching at the Henry Street House. The staff helped children get library cards for their public library and select appropriate books to check out. Younger children could read books from the small library at the Henry Street House, which was stocked particularly with the most popular fairy tales.[134] There were also many programs for older children.[135] Those between the ages fourteen and sixteen could receive a scholarship that supported them during a period of training for employment. Young women about to be married could attend classes on housekeeping and hygiene. Before the city recognized the need for special education services, the Henry Street House offered experimental classes for handicapped children.

More extensive action was to come. Wald successfully campaigned for what would become the federal Children's Bureau within the US Department of Labor. The idea for the bureau came to Wald in 1903, when she was reading the newspaper with a friend.[136] An article described a trip taken by the secretary of agriculture to check on the harm of the boll weevil to cotton crops in the South. Wald said, "If the Government can have a department to take such an interest in what is happening to the Nation's cotton crop, why can't it have a bureau to look after the Nation's crop of children?"[137] Later that year, Wald and a friend sent a telegram to President Teddy Roosevelt, who had visited the Henry Street House while serving years earlier as the New York City police commissioner. They asked to meet to discuss the idea of a children's bureau. Roosevelt replied immediately: "Bully. Come down and tell me about it."[138]

Creating the bureau took more time, nine years in all. In 1905, the National Child Labor Committee took a leadership role in lobbying for legislation, with the support of a diverse group of women's organizations.[139] After the usual drawn-out legislative battle, President Taft signed a bill in 1912 to create a bureau that would promote and advocate for child welfare. The Children's Bureau became the first government agency to focus specifically on the well-being of children and mothers. With initial funding of $25,640, Julia Lathrop, who had been active in the settlement movement, was appointed to run the agency. She became the first woman to head a federal bureau in the United States. Today, the Children's Bureau continues as part of the Department of Health and Human Services.

African Americans

Wald demonstrated her commitment to racial equality by hiring African American nurses and expanding settlement houses into African American neighborhoods. As mixing of the races was shocking at the time, African American nurses seldom treated white patients.[140] Wald still did what she could under these restrictions. The Henry Street House was open to African Americans, who regularly came as guests.[141] Wald "had no problem finding admirably trained and efficient" African American nurses and treating them as equals.[142] The Henry Street House would eventually employ twenty-five African American nurses.[143]

The first African American nurse Wald hired, Elizabeth Tyler, had the task of finding and helping the few and isolated African Americans in the nearby neighborhoods. Tyler was so effective that Edith Carter, a second African American nurse was hired.

New settlement house branches in African American neighborhoods in Manhattan's Upper West Side and North Harlem followed. The branches advocated for the rights of people of color as well as serving as community centers and health clinics.[144]

One action had a particularly important impact. The 1909 National Negro Conference held its opening reception at the Henry Street House.[145] Both whites and African Americans organized the gathering in response to race riots in 1908 in Springfield, Illinois, Abraham Lincoln's hometown. Organizers included national civil rights leaders, such as W. E. B. Du Bois, the renowned author and scholar, and Ida B. Wells, the journalist who had exposed the epidemic of lynching in the South. The leaders recognized the need for a national organization to promote equality of rights and eradicate racial discrimination. However, even in New York City, the location of the conference, few venues would host a mixed-race event. Wald stepped in to offer the Henry Street House. The meeting ultimately led to the founding of the National Association for the Advancement of Colored People, the influential civil rights organization.

Workers

Employers in New York City and elsewhere found immigrants to be an easily exploitable group. The large numbers with few if any specialized skills and a willingness to take any job they could find led to meager wages, grueling labor, and inhuman working conditions. In the garment industry that dominated the Lower East Side, women and children as well as men filled the jobs. Despite her privileged background, Wald considered herself a working woman and comrade to these workers.[146]

Always in the midst of social action in the city, Wald helped create the National Women's Trade Union League in 1903.[147] The union linked middle-class women and working women in an effort to eliminate sweatshop conditions. It supported worker strikes and campaigned for legislation to mandate an eight-hour workday. It was active at the time of a terrible tragedy in the city. In 1911, a fire at the Triangle Shirtwaist Factory in Greenwich Village killed 146 employees, including 123 women and girls. The fire still stands as the deadliest industrial disaster in American history. Most of the employees were Italian or Jewish immigrants, the youngest being two fourteen-year-old girls. In a four-year investigation, league members identified the conditions that led to the disaster and called for new workplace regulations.[148]

Decline of the Social Approach

Through the first two decades of the twentieth century, the Henry Street House and its public health model enjoyed considerable success. In 1911, a staff of fifty-five cared for 19,492 patients, made 175,953 home visits, and gave 18,934 first-aid treatments.[149] Looking back in 1934, Wald commented that the conditions she found in the Lower East Side when the Henry Street House opened had greatly improved.[150] The visiting nurses and other programs clearly met a need, and the demand for the program services extended well outside the area. With its success, the organization needed a clearly defined hierarchy and division of labor to ensure consistency in the programs. Communication became cumbersome.[151] By sheer force of personality, Wald managed to hold the enterprise together. But it would not last.

The 1920s saw a backlash emerge against the progressive views and policies of the previous several decades. A confluence of events made life difficult for organizations devoted to social justice. The revolution and Communist accession in Russia led many to accuse American socialists of sedition.[152] The Red Scare after

World War I focused on immigrants, who were often part of the labor movement and seen as anti-American. Laws restricting immigration followed. After winning the right to vote in 1920, the women's movement lost steam. At the same time, a more radical and adventuresome generation of young feminists viewed the domestic caring role that Wald and others embraced as outmoded.[153] More generally, Americans wanted what Republican president Warren Harding promised in 1920—a "return to normalcy." That promise meant replacing social experiments with complacency, collectivism with individualism, idealism with realism, and government action with private sector growth. Settlement homes were no longer compatible with the spirit of the 1920s.

Slowly but steadily, the changing times and generations marginalized the model of combining nursing and social work and the goal of reducing upstream sources of health inequality.[154] The Great Depression to follow in the 1930s raised the demand for health care and nursing, but other forces of change worked against the Henry Street House model. First, the growth of hospitals reduced the demand for visiting nurses.[155] Although once seen as places to avoid, hospitals had over the decades emerged as central to health care. Hospital care increasingly replaced home care as treatment protocols and surgical techniques advanced and as problems from chronic diseases gradually grew more common relative to the risks of death from infectious diseases. The work of nurses "reverted to a version of the support role they had provided to physicians in hospitals before their professionalization."[156] The nursing profession became increasingly technical, less present in the neighborhoods, and less focused on primary prevention.

For the Henry Street House, the hard times of the Great Depression and the loss of charitable backing meant salary cutbacks and competition for scarce resources.[157] Even the private insurance for home care that Metropolitan Life had originated eventually died out. The savings gained from home care fell as chronic illnesses became more prevalent and life-threatening acute illnesses receded. Policyholders preferred hospitals for treatment of serious illnesses, and payments to visiting nurses by Metropolitan Life and other insurance companies declined dramatically.[158] Families came to depend on prepaid health insurance policies to cover the costs of treatment and care rather than on life insurance policies.[159] Reimbursement under the health insurance policies was limited to treatments for specific health problems.[160] Benefits seldom covered the teaching, comforting, and relationship-building activities of the Henry Street House nurses.

While forces of change worked against the model of public health nursing that Wald had developed, her own health deteriorated.[161] She had purchased a home in Westport, Connecticut, to enjoy periods of respite from the hectic pace of the Henry Street House. In the 1920s, illness forced her to stay in Connecticut for long periods. In 1932, she was hospitalized for internal bleeding and anemia, and in 1933 she retired. A heart attack followed in 1937, and she died in 1940 at age seventy-three.

With Wald's retirement and death, internal friction at the Henry Street House undermined the tight connection that had existed between nursing and social work. Both occupations had become more professional and specialized than in the past, with each focused on its own areas of expertise.[162] Without Wald to hold things together by force of her talents and personality, a power struggle between the nursing and social work leaders resulted in a split. In 1944, the Visiting Nurse Service of New York became an independent agency that served the whole city, while the Henry Street House focused on social work in the Lower East Side.

A Return to Social Activism in Public Health Nursing?

Despite the changes that occurred after her retirement and death, Wald left an impressive legacy. Public health nursing has grown into a central part of the public health system, albeit in a different form than Wald envisioned. While John Snow ended up as an icon of public health after facing rejection and resistance to his ideas during his lifetime, Lillian Wald experienced the opposite. A successful and widely recognized leader during most of her life, she has been neglected as a public health founder in the decades that followed the Progressive Era. Recent calls to renew Wald's emphasis on social activism in public health, however, have enhanced her reputation.

As Wald would have hoped, public nursing today is a respected and thriving part of the nursing profession. The Association of Public Health Nurses notes that it constitutes "the largest segment of the professional public health workforce."[163] School nurses have a separate organization, the National Association of School Nurses, with more than seventeen thousand members and fifty affiliates. There is also the Association of Community Health Nursing Educators, and Public Health Nursing has its own member section in the American Public Health Association.

The diversity of activities and skills of public health nursing is striking. Public health nurses help pregnant women, infants and preschool-age children, schoolchildren and their families, and the disabled, elderly, and chronically ill. They work in schools, clinics, homes, and the community. Some focus on disease prevention, others on disease management, and still others on community health. Public health nursing has taken on new goals in dealing with problems of mental health, indigent populations, childhood immunizations, drug use, homelessness, disability, emergency preparedness, and health inequalities.[164] One can add to that list the goals of promoting lifestyle change to reduce risky sexual behavior, improve unhealthy diets, and encourage physical activity. Even home care has reemerged with funding from Medicare to care for the chronically ill.[165]

The split between public health nursing and social work would have saddened Wald, though both approaches have been successful on their own. The Henry Street House, now a social service organization, has "an expansive network of 18 facilities that deliver a wide range of social services, arts, and health care programs to more than 50,000 New Yorkers each year."[166] It primarily serves Asian, African American, and Latino residents rather than Jewish immigrants from Russia and Poland but still is devoted to helping disadvantaged groups.[167] The Visiting Nurse Service of New York, the other offspring of the Henry Street House, provides high-quality home and community health care to the city. It employs about thirteen thousand home health aides, nurses, rehabilitation therapists, clinicians, and social workers. On any given day it has nearly forty thousand patients. Much of the effort goes to helping the elderly, as the average age of the patients it serves is seventy-two.[168]

While Wald would be pleased and impressed by the expansion of public health nursing, she no doubt would be discouraged by the stubbornly persistent health inequalities in the United States. Despite some progress toward reducing these inequalities during Wald's time, most view current levels as unacceptably high and worsening. A recent review concludes that empirical research "yields a very persuasive finding of growing gaps in adult mortality and life expectancies across both education and income" in the United States but not in Europe or Canada.[169] In the United States, rising numbers of "deaths of despair" from suicide, drug abuse, alcoholism, and gun violence derive disproportionately from the less educated. Progress has occurred in reducing racial disparities in mortality, but whites still outlive African Americans by four years on average.[170]

Among its goals, public health nursing addresses problems of health inequality. Attentiveness to the health needs of an entire population, primary prevention, and community action requires responsiveness to disadvantaged groups whose health problems are generally the most serious. Nurses can provide cost-efficient community care for the most vulnerable. However, obstacles limit their effectiveness. There is concern that funding for public health nursing remains too low and that services are too fragmented.[171] The health care system tends to favor treatment over prevention and ability to pay over need. The public health struggle to improve the health of poor people—the driving ambition of Wald's life—continues today.

Several scholars and nurses have called to reinvigorate public health nursing so that it better matches Wald's original vision.[172] Some of what Wald advocated makes little sense today, particularly the domestic duties the nurses performed in cleaning and arranging the households of patients. Other activities remain critically relevant. Modern advocates of Wald's vision view as essential the nursing goals of providing comprehensive care, understanding the patient, and taking public responsibility for improving community social conditions Doing more to restore Wald's vision by addressing upstream, collective solutions is a fitting way to honor her accomplishments.

5.

The Social Epidemiologist
W. E. B. Du Bois, Racial Inequality, and Health

In 1896, several prominent and reform-minded Philadelphians expressed concern about the living conditions in a neighborhood not far from the city center. They deplored the disorder they saw—crime, disease, poverty—that was all too near their own homes. Susan Wharton, one of the city's philanthropists and part of the rich and prominent Quaker family that funded the Wharton School at the University of Pennsylvania, took charge.[1] She convinced the provost of the University of Pennsylvania, Charles Harrison, to sponsor a study of the neighborhood. They reasoned that a scientific study of the residents and their lives would identify ways to remedy the problems. Coming from the University of Pennsylvania, the findings of the study might have enough legitimacy to convince the often-corrupt city politicians to take some action.

The provost assigned a sociology professor at the University of Pennsylvania, Samuel Lindsay, to oversee the project and find a social scientist to carry out the research. A liberal fully committed to the project and its goal of helping those in need, Lindsay

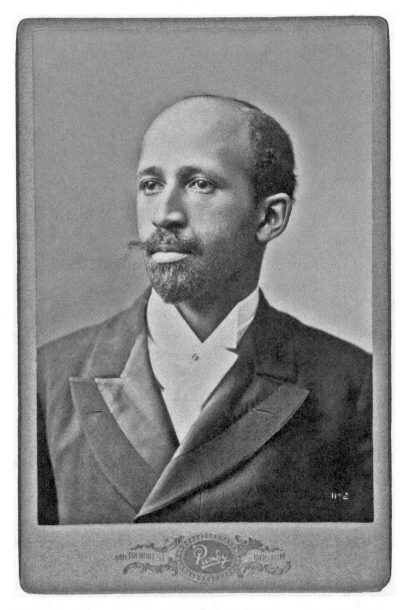

W. E. B. Du Bois, 1907. *Source*: Wikimedia Commons, by James E. Purdy, from the National Portrait Gallery, Washington, DC. Creative Commons CC0 1.0.

knew of an excellent choice for the job. The young man Lindsay had in mind brought superb qualifications. After receiving his undergraduate degree, he completed graduate degrees at Harvard and studied for two years with the leading social scientists in Germany—the center of intellectual life at the time. He was one of the most educated men in the country.[2] The young man was underemployed at the time and jumped at the chance to join the University of Pennsylvania. Lindsay hired him as an assistant instructor in sociology for one year, and the university paid his salary ($900) while he worked on the project.

The newly hired researcher moved into the neighborhood and began to gather data and interview residents. Through intense research and exceptional interpretative skills, and without the help of any university colleagues, he completed the study and would soon publish a 437-page book on the findings. The book was original, impressive in its research and scholarship, and offered new insights into the social problems of the neighborhood. Lindsay wrote that the work "proved to be far greater than our highest expectations."[3] After such an accomplishment, the University of Pennsylvania might be expected to offer a permanent position to such an outstanding scholar.

It was not to be, however. The promising candidate may have succeeded brilliantly in his education and writings, and he may have outshone other colleagues at the university, but it didn't matter. Something else prevented the hire: he was Black.

The scholar, W. E. B. Du Bois (pronounced dew-BOYS), had been hired to study a neighborhood consisting primarily of African Americans. He was tasked with understanding the source of the race problems in the city. Only an African American could live in the neighborhood, talk to the residents, and complete the study. It turned out, however, that the study did not discover what many Philadelphians had expected or wanted. He found that the social problems of poverty, violence, and poor health in the neighborhood resulted from an environment of racism and discrimination in the city and country. Du Bois focused more on the social organization of society than on the faults of individuals living in the neighborhood. He failed to confirm the prejudices held by most Americans.

Du Bois's book, *The Philadelphia Negro*, set a standard for a new type of social and epidemiological research. The work, seen as a founding text of what today is called social epidemiology, offered an innovative approach to public health and racial inequality in America.[4] Readers of the book today comment on the similarities between current race relations and the problems Du Bois described more than 120 years ago.[5] In good part thanks to Du Bois, however, the understanding we have of the influence of racism today contrasts strikingly with the views of racial inferiority and superiority held by most whites during his time. The inequalities have sadly persisted, but the explanations have changed radically.

Du Bois was a philosopher, historian, and sociologist by training and an activist and civil rights leader by choice. He became "the most prolific and, arguably, the most influential African American writer of his generation."[6] He had no connection to the established field of medicine or the newly emerging field of public health. Even today, few would classify him as a public health specialist. However, scholars have increasingly come to recognize the major contribution he made to public health in his studies of race.[7] One subdivision of public health, social epidemiology, investigates the "social determinants of population distributions of health, disease, and wellbeing, rather than treating such determinants as mere background to biomedical phenomena."[8] As Du Bois did, social epidemiology focuses on how the social organization of society and divisions based on social class, education, gender, race, ethnicity, and residence shape the distribution of health and disease.

The groundbreaking research and writings of W. E. B. Du Bois deserve attention in the history of public health. His work has not saved lives in the same way as that of other public health figures, but it did something of immense importance. It directed attention to the enduring problem of racial inequality as a source of disease, poor health, and premature death. Some offer the high praise of comparing Du Bois to John Snow. Both made lasting break-throughs in our understanding of the sources of human health.[9] But Du Bois stands out on his own for bringing racial justice to the forefront of public health.[10] Building on what Du Bois demonstrated more than 120 years ago, social epidemiology today has been "indelibly shaped by a concern over black/white differences in some fundamental health outcomes in the United States."[11]

Enduring Racial Inequality

Among the countless and shameful forms of mistreatment of African Americans in the United States, health disparities stand out. As Martin Luther King Jr. said, "Of all the forms of inequality, injustice in health is the most shocking and the most inhuman because it often results in physical death."[12] This shocking and in-human injustice has endured for over four hundred years of American history.[13] Never in the United States have African Americans experienced the same health as whites. Racial health disparities, so extreme during the long period of slavery, contin-ued after the Civil War. Even with freedom from slavery, the health problems of African Americans were so severe and so ob-vious that white experts tried to explain them away with claims of biological inferiority. In fact, though, the racial world that Du Bois would study in the 1890s had been brought about by a long history of mistreatment.

The Failure of Reconstruction

After the end of the Civil War and the immoral, brutal, and degrading period of slavery in the United States, there was hope that more equitable treatment of African Americans would follow. At first things looked promising. The period of Reconstruction in the South (1865-1877) sought to rehabilitate the southern states before they could rejoin the Union. Toward that end, Congress passed and the states ratified three constitutional amendments:

- Thirteenth Amendment: "Neither slavery nor involuntary servitude, except as a punishment for crime whereof the party shall have been duly convicted, shall exist within the United States, or any place subject to their jurisdiction."
- Fourteenth Amendment: No state shall "deny to any person within its jurisdiction the equal protection of the laws."
- Fifteenth Amendment: "The right of citizens of the United States to vote shall not be denied or abridged by the United States or by any State on account of race, color, or previous condition of servitude."

That the amendments became the law of the land was all the more impressive given the bitter resistance of opponents.

Northern Republicans expected the amendments to transform the South. Equal treatment of the races had become the law of the land, and military occupation of the former Confederate states by northern troops could enforce the law. The amendments certainly raised the hopes of African Americans for better lives, and initial progress promised still better things to come. Voters in the state of Mississippi elected Hiram Revels, an African American minister, to the Senate in 1870. He became the first African American to serve in Congress. Southern states elected several African American congressional representatives from 1869 onward. As a majority in some areas, African Americans took on local leadership roles that they had never enjoyed before. Although their power remained limited, the progress was encouraging.

Other federal legislation reinforced the constitutional amendments. Overriding President Andrew Johnson's veto, Congress established the Freedmen's Bureau to help formerly enslaved people in the transition to freedom. It did much good, at least initially. The bureau gave out food and clothing, helped legalize marriages and negotiate labor contracts between planters and field workers, and established new schools and hospitals.[14] In his overview of the benefits of Reconstruction, Du Bois pointed out that the Freedmen's Bureau helped to significantly extend education to African Americans. He said, "Seldom in the history of the world has an almost totally illiterate population been given the means of self-education in so short a time."[15]

The hopes for equality were never realized. Opposition to new policies and laws by southern whites and sympathetic northerners prevented real change. Whites found ways to get around the new amendments and laws. From the start, states and localities in the South passed "Black Codes" to restrict the freedom of formerly enslaved people. Vagrancy laws limited movement of workers and allowed authorities to arrest African Americans for minor violations (and then force them into involuntary work as prisoners). The codes restricted racial intermarriage, limited the right to own property, and replaced wage employment with apprenticeships. In another form of subjugation, African Americans ended up working as sharecroppers on land owned by whites rather than owning their own land. Sharecroppers paid rent in the form of crops but often stayed indebted to landowners and could barely survive on what they produced.

Demands of African Americans for better treatment were often met by violence. In 1866, for example, race riots in Memphis and New Orleans led to the deaths of dozens of African Americans and the burning of homes, churches, and schools. The Ku

Klux Klan, started in 1865 by ex-Confederate soldiers, used beatings, killings, lynchings, and intimidation against African Americans.

After a few years, support for Reconstruction and the commitment to racial equality began to wane. The Freedmen's Bureau, the source of much optimism, was often co-opted by local whites.[16] Its effectiveness diminished after only a few years, and it was abolished in 1872.[17] Worries about the corruption of newly elected officials in the South and disagreements about dealing with economic problems split the Republican Party on Reconstruction. Many in the North simply tired of the ongoing disorder in the South.[18] Perhaps returning control to the southern states would end the conflict and corruption. The issue came to a head after the disputed 1876 presidential election. When electoral votes in several states were contested and the victor was left unclear, the parties worked out a compromise. It gave the presidency to the Republican candidate in exchange for removing federal troops and ending federal interference in the southern states. In the end, whites maintained their domination in the South.

Southern and Northern Segregation

With the end of Reconstruction and the return of home rule to southern states, a fully developed system of segregation called Jim Crow emerged. Jim Crow was a name given to an African American character created by a white actor during the time of slavery. The character portrayed African Americans in racist ways, and the term came to refer to the system of laws and behavioral norms requiring the segregation of African Americans and whites. An 1890 law in Louisiana compelled African Americans to ride in separate rail cars from whites. Other state laws required different schools, hotels, drinking fountains, and public restrooms. Where full physical separation of the races was not possible, as on buses, in restaurants, and in stores, separate seating areas or entrances were set aside for African Americans.

Parts of the system circumvented the right to vote given by the Fifteenth Amendment. State and local laws required ownership of property, proof of literacy, or payment of a tax. Some places instituted "grandfather clauses" that allowed citizens to avoid these barriers if they could prove that their grandfathers had been eligible to vote—an impossibility for African Americans, whose grandfathers had been enslaved. The laws applied equally to whites and African Americans but affected only African Americans. This sort of legislation worked efficiently, systematically disfranchising African Americans throughout the South.

The restrictions appeared to violate the constitutional mandates for equal protection under the law and the right to vote. However, the 1896 Supreme Court decision in *Plessy v. Ferguson* allowed Jim Crow laws to continue under a standard that separate but equal facilities met constitutional requirements. The laws thus remained in place until overturned in 1954 with the court's ruling in *Brown v. Board of Education*. Not until the protests led by Martin Luther King Jr. and many other civil rights leaders and the passage of the Civil Rights Act of 1964 did legally mandated segregation in the southern states begin to disappear.

The prospects for improved health and quality of life of African Americans in the South were never realized. For the 90 percent of the 6.5 million African Americans living in the South, mostly in rural areas, daily life meant poverty, hard work, and poor nutrition.[19] Child mortality was high, and adults struggled to survive. In 1890, African Americans could expect on average to live only thirty-five and a half years.[20]

With continued mistreatment in the South, many African Americans migrated to northern cities looking for work and a better life. They found segregation to be the norm. Whites and African Americans typically lived in separate neighborhoods and attended different schools. Employers kept the best jobs for whites, and African American opportunities were restricted to manual labor, servant and cleaning roles in white households, or professional, shopkeeping, and craft jobs that served other African Americans.[21] As only a small part of the population in most cities, African Americans had little political power, even with the right to vote.[22] Poverty and deprivation remained much higher among them than among whites.

Northern segregation damaged the health of African Americans in innumerable ways, much as it did in the South. Residents lacked nutritious food, did not have access to the same medical care as whites, lived in the most disease-filled parts of cities, and faced debilitating struggles of dealing with poverty and discrimination. Such was the world Du Bois confronted when he began his study in Philadelphia. He would be the first to demonstrate through empirical study how the social conditions of deprivation contributed to the poor health and well-being of African Americans.

One of the Most Educated Men in America

A Happy and Unusual African American Childhood

William Edward Burghardt Du Bois was born in 1868, only three years after the end of the Civil War, in Great Barrington, a small farming community in western Massachusetts. Although slavery had ended only a few years earlier, it did not directly affect his childhood. On his mother's side, his great-grandfather Tom had been brought to America and enslaved but received his freedom after fighting in the Revolutionary War.[23] He took his last name, Burghardt, from the white family that enslaved him until his freedom. His descendants had lived for generations in Great Barrington and its environs. On his father's side, the Du Bois name traced back to a white French father and African American mother. The children of the couple were born in the Caribbean but later resettled in New York State.[24]

When Alfred Du Bois came to Great Barrington in 1867, he met Mary Burghardt, now thirty-five years old.[25] They married, having one son who was called Willie until college.[26] Alfred Du Bois soon left to find a new home for the family in Connecticut, but Mary preferred to stay with her family in Great Barrington, and the husband and wife never reunited.[27] With the help of her relatives, Mary raised her son in the town of about four thousand residents.[28] Unlike the South and large cities of the North, Great Barrington enjoyed civil relations between whites and Blacks.[29] Class and income appeared more important, as newly arrived Irish immigrants, rather than long-established African Americans, faced the most severe prejudice.[30]

Du Bois lived, in his own words, a sheltered and happy childhood. Although poor, he had sufficient food, shelter, and clothing, and he never felt that others looked down on him for his family's lack of money.[31] To the contrary, he so excelled in school as to be seen as a village prodigy.[32] He became a favorite of the teachers and gained the respect of other students. Perhaps more surprising, he felt little in the way of discrimination from white classmates:

> I had, as a child, almost no experience of segregation or color discrimination. My schoolmates were invariably white; I joined quite naturally all games, excursions, church festivals; recreations like coasting, swimming, hiking and games. I was in and out of the homes of nearly all my mates, and ate and played with them. I was as a boy long unconscious of color discrimination in any obvious and specific way.[33]

Only in high school did he begin to feel the pressure of racial distinction.[34] Even then, he felt more disdain for the few who snubbed him than shame about his race. He had confidence in his abilities to outdo others and expected to be treated fairly.

It is no wonder that Du Bois developed strong feelings of confidence that would guide him throughout his life. The combination of a quick mind, an endless capacity for hard work, and ambition to excel was exceptional by any standard. His reserved, dignified, and somewhat formal manner similarly impressed others.[35] He did so well in school that a white principal wanted him to take college prep courses. With such encouragement, Du Bois aimed high—he wanted to attend Harvard.[36] After graduating from high school, the only African American in his class,[37] local churches and white supporters helped fund his enrollment at Fisk University, a private, historically African American university in Nashville, Tennessee. Fisk was not Harvard, but as one of several universities founded after the Civil War to educate freed people, it had its attractions for Du Bois. Having been sheltered in Great Barrington, he looked forward to exploring an exciting new world, one where he would meet other African Americans from altogether different backgrounds than his own.[38]

The Shock of Segregation

At age seventeen and naive about racial relations in most of the country, Du Bois was amazed by what he saw in Nashville. He was impressed by the rich diversity among African Americans.[39] He was also disturbed by something equally new—white hostility and the mistreatment of African Americans. His sheltered upbringing in Great Barrington did not prepare him for the world of racism he now experienced. Being educated and from a middle-class background provided no buffer to the racism experienced by less privileged African Americans. "Lynching was a continuing and recurrent horror during my college days: from 1885 through 1894, 1,700 Negroes were lynched in America. Each death was a scar upon my soul."[40] He further wrote, "No one but a Negro going into the South without previous experience of color caste can have any conception of its barbarism."[41] He soon developed a "belligerent attitude" toward segregation and adopted a newfound identification with his race.[42]

Despite the race problems outside the university, Du Bois enjoyed college and completed his undergraduate degree in only three years. He continued to excel academically, although teachers recognized some conceit to go along with his intelligence.[43] He admitted to being sharp-tongued,[44] and his formal manner and lack of easy comradery made him appear to be remote and arrogant to some.[45] Overall, however, Du Bois viewed his time at Fisk with fondness.[46] The university offered a strong if basic curriculum, gave him the opportunity to edit a university literary magazine, and reinforced his ambition to continue his education at Harvard.

With help from his Fisk professors and support from an educational foundation, Du Bois was, somewhat surprisingly given the racism of the period, accepted by Harvard University.[47] He began there after graduating from Fisk in 1888. Although he already had an undergraduate degree, Harvard enrolled him as a junior, and he soon obtained his second bachelor's degree. Segregation in the Boston area differed from that in Nashville. It was present but not legally mandated. He lived in an off-campus rooming house owned by an African American woman and found companionship with other African Americans, often outside the university.[48] Du Bois avoided much of the discrimination by focusing on his studies in a "self-imposed segregation."[49] He had little contact with white students outside of class.[50] His personality may have struck others as standoffish, but avoiding undergraduate activities limited the enmity and rejection he would face. He would say, "I was in Harvard, but not of it."[51]

As he had done all his life, Du Bois performed exceptionally well in school and enjoyed the atmosphere of intellectuality. Majoring in philosophy, he studied with William James, the country's premier philosopher. He graduated cum laude in two years and was selected as one of six commencement speakers.[52] During that time, Du Bois became interested in sociology and race issues. Wanting in particular to investigate the American slave trade, he made plans to enter graduate school. Thanks to a fellowship, he continued his education in Harvard's graduate program in the social sciences. He received a master's degree and began a project on the failed efforts to suppress the African slave trade in America. The research would become his doctoral thesis.[53]

Still not yet satisfied with his achievements, Du Bois sought to extend his education in the social sciences by studying in Europe. The best universities in the world at the time were in Germany. Du Bois managed, despite some resistance to his application from foundation leaders, to obtain funding to support his study at the University of Berlin.[54] There he learned about newly developing social science research methods that emphasized objective, scientific observation and data gathering. He developed "an almost blind faith in science and a determination to engage in a career of research, writing, and teaching."[55]

Living in Germany brought new insights about race as well as research. Much as he had been shocked by the brutalities of segregation in the South, Du Bois was now shocked by the fair and respectful treatment that he received in Germany. Whites there showed little sign of prejudice toward him. He was treated as a privileged student and regarded with respect rather than hostility.[56] His treatment in Germany proved that race relations need not take the form they did in the United States.

Returning to the United States in 1894 again brought back the realities of segregation. Du Bois would soon finish his dissertation and receive a PhD in history from Harvard. With degrees from Harvard plus years of study in Berlin, Du Bois was one of the most educated men in the country. In 1895, he became the first African American to obtain a doctorate from Harvard in any field.[57] It is hard to exaggerate the accomplishment this degree represented. Doctoral degrees were rare at the time for people of any race, and Du Bois had overcome much to reach his goal. As one expert summarizes, "In a land where most of the nine million people of African descent were a generation removed from centuries of enslavement, where literacy was in many places a near capital offense for these people, W.E.B. Du Bois had become one of the most intellectually credentialed men, Black or White, in the United States."[58]

By all rights, given his accomplishments, prestigious universities should have been clamoring to hire him as a professor. Du Bois soon realized, however, that white universities and colleges had no interest in inviting him to join the faculty.[59] He instead wrote letters to historically African American universities and gratefully accepted the first offer he received. Wilberforce University, a religious school for African Americans in Ohio, offered him a position to teach Latin and Greek. From the start, he fit poorly in the school. He wanted to teach sociology rather than classics, objected to the low academic standards, and felt uncomfortable with the religious atmosphere.[60] With well-justified feelings of intellectual superiority, he urged Wilberforce leaders—sometimes quite bluntly—to adopt his ideals for a university.[61] Even his appearance on campus, which in the tradition of a German gentleman sometimes included a cane and white gloves, set him apart from colleagues and administrators.[62] He stayed at Wilberforce for two years (1894–1896). Despite the happy events of getting married and receiving his PhD from Harvard during that time, he was miserable. Staying there longer meant "spiritual death."[63]

A Social Perspective on Racial Inequality

The offer from the University of Pennsylvania—to carry out a study of an African American neighborhood in Philadelphia while working for the university—came out of the blue. It felt like salvation to Du Bois. Here was a chance to apply the new social science research methods he had learned to a problem of personal and public importance. And he would be part of a prestigious university where colleagues shared his intellectual ideals and devotion to knowledge.

He soon felt the sting of second-class treatment, however. Despite his superb qualifications, his appointment was to last only one year. It came with the denigrating title of assistant instructor. He later wrote, "I was given no real academic standing, no office at the University, no official recognition of any kind; my name was eventually omitted from the catalogue; I had no contact with students, and very little with members of the faculty, even in my own department."[64] Regular contact with Lindsay, whom he always remembered warmly, was the only link to the university. As would become even more apparent over time, the university viewed him as expendable.[65] Du Bois would resent the unfairness for the rest of his life.

Thinking Wrong about Race

As he planned his research, Du Bois began to better appreciate the underlying agenda of the sponsors of the study—Wharton, Harrison, and Lindsay. They viewed Philadelphia as one of the most corrupt cities in the country and, somewhat idealistically, hoped to reform its government. In their view, the burdens placed on the African American community made up a major part of the challenges that the city needed to address. A first step toward reform would come from a scientifically documented study of the social conditions of African American Philadelphians. Du Bois, of course, was equally committed to the application of scientific methods to social problems, but he cared less about the politics behind his appointment.[66] He had a grander vision than to help the city reformers. He saw the opportunity to help African Americans in the city by not only describing the problems but also by identifying the causes of the problems.

A key part of that goal was to show that "the world was thinking wrong about race."[67] White stereotypes wrongly viewed African Americans as a homogenous group of inferiors rather than a diverse group beleaguered by an all-encompassing racism. At the time, social Darwinism dominated popular theories of race differences. Using an evolutionary analogy, social Darwinism viewed differences across social groups as the result of a process of survival of the fittest that was akin to the process of natural selection in Darwin's theory. A disadvantaged position in the world of social competition demonstrated, according to the theory, poor fitness for survival in a modernizing, industrializing economy. The hierarchy of races thus reflected the natural order of society.

Du Bois rejected pseudobiological theories, which he properly viewed as racist and unscientific. A scientific study would debunk the evolutionary claims of his opponents.[68] It would help show that the problems of African Americans in the city were symptoms rather than causes of racial inequality.[69] This insight would begin to transform thinking about how social conditions shaped disparities in human health. It would also produce what later scholars called a masterpiece of social science research.[70]

A John Snow–Like Commitment to High-Quality Research Methods

Du Bois and his wife moved into a one-room apartment in the middle of Philadelphia's Seventh Ward, the neighborhood to be the subject of his research. In his words, "We lived there a year, in the midst of an atmosphere of dirt, drunkenness, poverty, and crime."[71] At the time, Philadelphia was the country's second-largest city and home to the largest African American population outside the South.[72] The city's rapid growth after the Civil War brought both extraordinary progress and unexpected challenges. The Seventh Ward revealed the gap between the progress and challenges in concrete form. The expansive homes of distinguished and rich white families in the ward displayed the progress enjoyed by one segment of the city, while the nearby dilapidated housing of impoverished African Americans made visible the challenges in meeting the needs of the less fortunate parts of the district.[73]

Du Bois faced a daunting task. How much could a lone researcher do to capture the diversity and complexity of the neighborhood? He had to gather, organize, and analyze data, go house-to-house to interview residents, observe the activities in the streets, monitor the comings and goings at local bars and gambling houses, master the historical record of the city, use information from recent national censuses, create meticulous maps of the conditions of each block, and learn about the physical environment of buildings, streets, and homes.[74] He wanted to learn of the location, work, homes, and daily activities of the African Americans in the neighborhood. Above all, he wanted to understand their relations with white fellow citizens.[75] Everything had to be done systematically and carefully in order to make a convincing case for the study's conclusions.

Neighborhood residents did not make his job easy. Du Bois would say that they "received me with no open arms. They had a natural dislike to being studied like a strange species."[76] Imagine the unusual appearance of an African American dressed in suit and bow tie knocking on the doors in the poorest streets of the city and speaking to often illiterate residents in a formal, educated manner. Yet, through unceasing effort, Du Bois managed to personally visit and talk with five thousand people.[77] He spent much time in libraries as well. He completed all this work so thoroughly that he could say in hindsight that his methods and findings had "withstood the criticism of 60 years."[78] All in all, it was a "prodigious display of sociological detective work."[79]

The hard work and state-of-the art empirical investigation served as an implicit criticism of white scholars who all too willingly jumped to conclusions about African Americans from the shallowest of evidence. He challenged these armchair theorists who had little contact with people and their social worlds.[80] Interviewing, talking to, and observing people in real life would make it easy to dismiss broad conjectures about race. As Du Bois would say, "a slum is not a simple fact," but a symptom that required detailed study.[81] Accurately describing residents in the neighborhood could be painful. He would see up close the suffering, desperation, and deprivation of African Americans and the smug rationalizations of whites about their conduct toward them. Nonetheless, he faced this unpleasantness without turning aside.

One can see some parallels between John Snow's groundbreaking epidemiological studies of cholera and Du Bois's early social epidemiology. Snow identified unsanitary water as the root cause of cholera outbreaks, while Du Bois identified "systemic inequality of racism as the root cause of diseases and deaths in the 7th Ward in Philadelphia."[82] Both Snow and Du Bois used maps, statistics, and shoe leather to draw reliable conclusions.[83] Both were highly educated men who were strongly committed to the scientific method, although Snow was able to use natural experiments in ways that Du Bois could not. Sharon Jones-Eversley and Lorraine Dean argue that, given the parallels of their research methods, Du Bois should be recognized, as Snow has been, as a founder of modern epidemiology.[84]

Health and Mortality

The careful presentation of death rates in *The Philadelphia Negro* demonstrated a substantial African American disadvantage. In the Seventh Ward, the annual death rate for African Americans, 30.5 deaths per 1,000 people, exceeded the death rate of whites, 24.3 deaths per 1,000 people, by 20 percent.[85] If African Americans had shared the same death rate as whites, about one out of every five of those who died each year would have lived longer. Who was at most risk of dying? The race gap was largest and the rates of African American deaths highest among infants and among men. The major causes of death among African Americans were consumption (tuberculosis), pneumonia, heart disease, and stillbirths. Du Bois astutely noted that the situation was actually worse than the statistics indicated. The African American community had many more young people and women than the white population. As those two groups typically had low death rates, the composition of the population hid some of the African American disadvantage.[86]

A clear correlation existed between the poor health of African Americans in the Seventh Ward and their environment. African Americans lived in the unhealthiest parts and worst housing in the neighborhood.[87] At the time, only about 14 percent of the families in the Seventh Ward had flush toilets and running water. At the other extreme, 20 percent had no private yard and no private outhouse.[88] Many parts of the neighborhood were littered with garbage.[89] The poor sanitation and its undeniable connection to health problems appeared similar to those in London that Chadwick had described more than fifty years earlier.

Other evidence further confirmed that the higher African American death rate largely resulted from living conditions.[90] Du Bois pointed to the fact that African American death rates outside the Seventh Ward varied widely. The worst African American slum in Philadelphia, the Fifth Ward, had the worst sanitation and an extremely high death rate.[91] In contrast, the most affluent African American part of the city, the Thirtieth Ward, had good houses, clean streets, and a low death rate. The Seventh Ward fell between these two extremes. It was a mistake of logic, although one made all too often, to assume that living conditions were the same for whites and African Americans and that disparities in health and mortality resulted from the poor habits of African Americans.[92] The disparities instead pointed to the disadvantaged living conditions of African Americans in the city.

About seven years later, in 1906, Du Bois published a report using statistics for the country as a whole rather than for one city. It strengthened the findings in *The Philadelphia Negro*. He reported that annual death rates in areas of the United States with adequate reporting systems were 30.2 deaths per 1,000 people for African Americans and 17.3 deaths per 1,000 people for whites.[93] The huge racial gap was accompanied by variation across the country. Death rates for African Americans were lower in northern than southern cities.[94] For example, the African American annual death rate of 46.7 deaths per 1,000 people in Charleston, South Carolina, contrasted with the annual death rate of 18.0 deaths per 1,000 people in Cleveland.[95] He further noted that whites living in the disease-prone areas near the Chicago stockyards had a higher death rate than African Americans in other parts of the city. Racial traits and tendencies could not account for this variation.[96] Du Bois reasoned that if social and economic conditions were the same, racial differences in sickness and death would be nearly eliminated.[97]

Specific recommendations to deal with the poor health of African Americans followed from the findings.[98] Du Bois called for better sanitation, efforts to stamp out consumption, and greater access to hospitals, physicians, and nursing. Special attention should be given to proper care for pregnant women and children. Organizing local health leagues to disseminate information on healthy practices would help. If carried out, these changes would steadily reduce high African American mortality until it reached levels typical among whites.

After presenting the facts, Du Bois sought to convince his white readers that improving the health of African Americans was not only possible but to their benefit. The poor health of African Americans limited the workforce, placed a burden on the community and its charities, and required a greater commitment of medical resources.[99] Such disparities should spur leaders to do more to help rather than find excuses to do nothing. He noted, "There have, for instance, been few other cases in the history of civilized peoples where human suffering has been viewed with such peculiar indifference."[100]

Diversity among African Americans

While identifying the disparities in health and well-being between African Americans and whites, Du Bois emphasized what can be seen as a breakthrough in thinking about race: the African American community was heterogeneous and diversified rather than monolithic.[101] He verified what should have been obvious, that a class hierarchy existed among African Americans as it existed among whites. An emerging African American middle class of professionals, merchants, and small business owners had resources that low-wage workers and the unemployed did not. Class differences among African Americans as well as between races affected health and well-being. If middle-class African Americans lived healthy lives similar to those of whites, it implied that bettering the living conditions of lower-class African Americans would improve their health. This finding contradicted racist stereotypes that ignored the accomplishments of middle-class African Americans.

Along with class, diversity among African Americans related in good part to migration status. The vast differences between the longer-term African American residents of Philadelphia and the new migrants from the rural South resulted in health differences. About one-half of the residents of the Seventh Ward were born in the South.[102] The most recent migrants had settled in the least expensive areas in slums and were exposed to the worst health conditions.[103] In contrast, African Americans with established roots in the city managed to do better. They were better educated and sometimes even wealthy and did not conform to white stereotypes of backwardness. The advantaged class was small, but the robust health of its members contrasted with that of new migrants to the city.

Du Bois used maps in ways that illustrated the gaps in social position both between and within racial groups. Inequalities in health and well-being had a spatial pattern that reflected segregation in living arrangements. His hand-drawn maps of blocks located in the Seventh Ward coded the race and class of residents in the dwellings and required meticulous care and detailed knowledge of the neighborhood's inhabitants. The clustering of the light and dark markings visually revealed that whites separated themselves from African Americans and middle-class African Americans separated themselves from lower-class African Americans.[104] In terminology used today, the patterns portrayed the intersection of race and class.

The Social Sources of Racial Inequality

The Burden of History

It made little sense to Du Bois, a trained historian, to describe the current health conditions of African Americans without exploring the long-term course of events that led to the conditions. *The Philadelphia Negro* offers a detailed overview of the history of African Americans in the city. One general pattern of change tended to repeat itself: periods of progress and raised hopes were invariably followed by a resurgence of racism that reasserted white dominance.

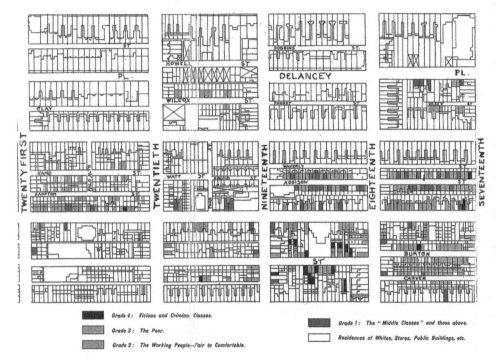

Grade 4: Vicious and Criminal Classes.

Grade 3: The Poor.

Grade 2: The Working People--Fair to Comfortable.

Grade 1: The "Middle Classes" and those above.

Residences of Whites, Stores, Public Buildings, etc.

Detail of Du Bois's map of the Seventh Ward from *The Philadelphia Negro* (1899), showing segregation by race and class. *Source*: Wikimedia Commons, from Widener Library, Harvard University.

Around the time of the American Revolution, the African American population in Philadelphia was small. Although most often brought to the city enslaved, African Americans benefited from antislavery views of the public. The state of Pennsylvania passed a law in 1780 that prohibited slavery for children born to enslaved people and gradually emancipated those already in slavery.[105] With new freedoms and the settlement of people who escaped slavery in the South, the population of African Americans grew to about 10 percent of the city's population. Many freed people learned trades, and others worked for wages as servants. New schools and churches for African Americans created feelings of belongingness.[106] The general outlook was encouraging.

During the 1820s to the 1840s, however, the growth of manufacturing in the city created new conflicts. The manufacturing jobs attracted white immigrants who competed with African Americans for work.[107] The threat of African American workers exacerbated racial hostilities among lower-class whites. From 1829 to 1842, a series of race riots occurred in which white mobs assaulted, beat, and killed African Americans, looted their homes, and burned down buildings.[108] The violence ended in 1842 after the local militia was called out by the mayor to restore order. With the new wave of violence, intimidation, and discrimination, the social position and economic well-being of African Americans in the city deteriorated.

After the Civil War, the African American population grew modestly but much more slowly than the white population.[109] With whites dominating manufacturing jobs, African Americans managed to find niche employment as artisans, caterers, and self-employed business owners.[110] Again, however, prospects for wider prosperity were ended by external events. Beginning in 1870 and continuing with the failures of Reconstruction, freed people from the South accounted for a mass migration to Philadelphia. An influx of fifteen thousand African American migrants, most from rural areas of Maryland, Virginia, and North Carolina, overwhelmed African American neighborhoods.[111] The efforts in the South to prevent freed people from bettering themselves meant that the new urban migrants were untrained, poorly educated, and unfamiliar with city life. They did not mix well with whites or the settled African Americans who had made some modest progress over the decades. As corrupt officials exploited African Americans to obtain their votes, racial tensions rose again.

Given the racial animus created by the competition for jobs plus the influx of freed people unprepared for city life, many African Americans lived in deprived circumstances and suffered from poor health. Knowing where African Americans came from and what forces had over the decades placed them at such a disadvantage was crucial. But more was needed beyond history. Du Bois wanted to show how employment discrimination and white prejudice shaped the daily lives of African Americans currently in the Seventh Ward. He would supply an insightful and discouraging narrative.

White Prejudice and Employment Discrimination

By 1896, when Du Bois started his research, the burden of slavery had left African Americans in vulnerable positions in the city. As in the past, white prejudice was a ubiquitous and unavoidable force in the lives of African Americans.[112] The African Americans interviewed by Du Bois regarded "prejudice as the chief cause of their present unfortunate condition."[113] Du Bois was careful not to attribute all African American problems to white prejudice. Rather, in understated and careful wording, he said that white prejudice was a "far more powerful social force than most Philadelphians realize."[114]

The attention to white prejudice and discrimination makes clear that Du Bois was presenting more than a study of African Americans.[115] His was a study of human relationships, of the social divide between whites and African Americans—what he called the color line. It was an apt metaphor. The color line obstructed African Americans, even those highly trained, from obtaining good jobs. Other than the small numbers of middle-class professionals and business owners, most African Americans could hope only for transient jobs or domestic service. It was not possible to join a trade union, work in an office, or supervise whites.[116]

To complement the statistics, Du Bois described personal accounts of discrimination obtained from his interviews. One African American born in Jamacia had a successful career as a mechanic in England, but after coming to Philadelphia, he was told that despite his skills he could not be hired because others would not work with him. After two years of searching, he ended up working odd jobs as a laborer.[117] Another African American with light skin had worked in a tailor shop for three weeks and by all accounts his work was acceptable. When it became known that he was African American, other tailors refused to work with him, and he was fired.[118] One young African American woman was hired for temporary work as a servant. Her mistress wanted to keep her on permanently but could not because all the other servants were white.[119]

Even those who, like Du Bois, were highly educated had little opportunity to utilize their talents. Du Bois recounts the story of an African American who graduated from the University of Pennsylvania with a degree in mechanical engineering. He was hired as an engineer through a job advertisement but was fired after only a few hours of work when the employer discovered that he was Black. Du Bois noted with irony that the engineer ended up working as a waiter at the University Club, "where his white fellow graduates dine."[120] Given the gap between his own educational credentials and his job, Du Bois may well have identified with the engineer.

Employment restrictions placed on African Americans often had a financial basis. White workers and trade union members benefited from restricting competition.[121] Employers did not often publicly declare their intent to discriminate—race was seldom listed as a formal job requirement, as it might be in the South. But less blatant discrimination occurred. It was easy for employers to say that they would lose customers and workers from integration or to rely on crude stereotypes about the inadequate qualifications of African Americans. With fewer chances for work, African Americans were forced to accept low wages. The employers who did hire them often took advantage of the circumstance by paying them less than whites.[122]

White immigration contributed to the employment discrimination against African Americans. Formerly enslaved people who came to Philadelphia had no experience in an industrial urban setting and little training to aid them in manufacturing work. They were unaccustomed to freedom and unfamiliar with the particulars of wage employment. The waves of white immigrants not only enjoyed the advantages of white skin and more positive attitudes of white employers, but in competition for low-wage jobs, their experiences with freedom also gave them "a powerful advantage over the recently freed slaves."[123]

A few employers showed that it was possible to overcome white prejudice in hiring African Americans. It required resistance to public opinion, however. One owner of a cabinet-making factory trained the son of a long-term African American porter at the company to learn the trade. Although the other workers objected strenuously, the employer stood firm. At the time of the interview, the young man had worked at the company for seven years. Du Bois included other isolated examples of an African American chemist and an African American jeweler who worked successfully for white employers.[124] Such employment was rare, however. Du Bois complained in asking, "How long can a city teach its black children that the road to success is to have a white face?"[125]

Du Bois noted that prejudice and discrimination particularly harmed African American women. Suffering from both racism and sexism, their job prospects were even bleaker than those of men.[126] He estimated that about 66 percent of African American women in Philadelphia worked—and they certainly needed the income.[127] The first edition of the book included a special report on domestic work written by a student and colleague, Isabel Eaton. With the same careful attention to data and methods as Du Bois employed, she reported that 91 percent of African American working women in Pennsylvania were employed in domestic service.[128] The work was poorly paid, often boring, and viewed as lowly, but African American women had few other choices.

Consequences of Blocked Opportunities

The mistreatment of African Americans in the labor market had implications for health. The lack of work and income meant living in unsanitary conditions and lacking nutritious food. As Du Bois stated, "bad ventilation, lack of outdoor life for women and children, poor protection against dampness and cold are undoubtedly the chief causes of the excessive death rate."[129]

The insidious consequences of mistreatment went well beyond health. Du Bois included chapters on illiteracy, crime, pauperism, alcoholism, and family breakup that described the problems of the Seventh Ward in much detail. African Americans naturally felt frustrated and demoralized when told that success came from honesty, efficiency, and talent but then saw those claims violated by prejudice and discrimination in their own lives. Why seek jobs or advancement that, based on race alone, would never come?[130] Some of the least advantaged African Americans, particularly new arrivals from the South whose opportunities for even menial work were few, resorted to crime. Furthermore, the lack of jobs and money led to family instability.

Well-to-do white Philadelphians sometimes believed that, although they could not employ African Americans, they could ease their conscience with charitable work and contributions. Du Bois argued that white benevolence helped little. Most charities in the city restricted their aid to whites.[131] That part of charitable donations going to the African American community did little to address the underlying source of the problems. The best way for whites to aid African American citizens would be to employ workers according to ability, offer training to raise that ability, and educate boys and girls to prepare them for meaningful and steady employment.[132]

A Dual Appeal

White readers could not mistake the key theme of *The Philadelphia Negro* that the most powerful forces behind the problems of African Americans were white prejudice and employment discrimination. Du Bois drew out the obvious recommendation from his insights. Simply put, whites should stop discrimination because it "is morally wrong, politically dangerous, industrially wasteful, and socially silly."[133] Having created the social conditions in which African Americans found themselves living, the white community had a duty to help rectify the wrongs. Du Bois appealed to whites in arguing it was to the advantage of all that the "two races should strive side by side to realize the ideals of the republic and make this truly a land of equal opportunity for all men."[134] He emphasized that efforts to guarantee equality were in the best interests of whites and the city overall.[135]

Du Bois had recommendations for African Americans as well. They should protest injustice but also strive for self-improvement. Reflecting his own Victorian upbringing, Du Bois called for African Americans to establish stronger, more stable families.[136] They should direct efforts to lessening idleness and crime and adopt values of discipline and hard work.[137] He also called for the most successful African Americans to help others of their race, to take on a stronger leadership role in the community.[138] All African Americans would benefit from recognizing their common interests and joining together to improve social conditions.

Descriptions of the failings of Africans Americans in the lower and middle classes and calls for personal changes in behavior sound moralistic and judgmental today.[139] Scholars see elitism in his desires for African Americans to live up to the values of the white middle class.[140] Du Bois's biographer, David Levering Lewis, called the book a "great, schizoid monograph" in its dual appeal to whites and blacks.[141] The appeal to whites included criticisms of African Americans and emphasized reform rather than transformation. Du Bois himself would later reject the reformism he advocated early on by recognizing the need for wholesale changes in the structure of the economy and society.

Despite these weaknesses, *The Philadelphia Negro* was, in the words of Lewis, "a breakthrough achievement, a virtually solitary departure from the hereditarian theorizing of the times."[142] Rejection of these theories was a precondition for eliminating racial differences and making integration possible.[143] Du Bois "relentlessly reminded his readers that race and racism distorted and deformed African American social development."[144] It is hard to downplay the importance of treating race differences in health and well-being as the consequence of social conditions, the history of servitude, and discrimination in the labor market.

At the time of its 1899 publication, *The Philadelphia Negro* received respectful reviews. Some journals and magazines ignored the book altogether, but others praised it for the careful and objective examination of data and the sympathetic treatment of African Americans.[145] Even the popular press, including well-known magazines such as the *Nation, Literary Digest*, the *Yale Review*, and several African American publications, praised the book.[146] In hindsight, however, the work failed to gain the recognition it deserved. The country simply wasn't ready to reject its racist beliefs and behaviors. It would take decades of additional research combined with social activism and legal challenges to make the theme of the study more tolerable to social scientists and the public more generally. *The Philadelphia Negro* is one of those initially unappreciated books that "has grown markedly in influence a century after its initial publication."[147]

That statement certainly applies to public health. Although Du Bois helped spawn "a whole new field of research,"[148] the approach would not be accepted quickly. Eventually, his work would help transform the way the field of public health treats race.[149]

A Life of Activism

For the rest of his long life, Du Bois would look back on *The Philadelphia Negro* with pride. He knew that few people ever read the long and detailed volume, but he was consoled by the respect it received.[150] That meant little in January 1898, however, when his appointment at the University of Pennsylvania ended.[151] He left with bitterness over the unwillingness of the university to offer even minimal recognition for his scholarship with an extension of his temporary instructorship.[152] Despite the slight, he knew he had done something special with his research. Why not extend the perspective on race and the high-quality research methods used successfully in Philadelphia to other parts of the country? He could demonstrate, as he had in Philadelphia, that absent white prejudice and discrimination, African Americans had the capability to become equal citizens in America.[153] He would continue to rely on facts, measurements, and research that ultimately would help change society.[154] This program of research guided his work for more than the next decade of his life.

The plan would not be carried out at the University of Pennsylvania or any other similar university. Race restricted the choices for a professorship.[155] Du Bois therefore accepted a position at an all-African American institution, Atlanta University. The university leaders there recognized the value of the research Du Bois had done and shared his goal of racial equality. They encouraged him to develop his program for the social scientific study of African Americans and to lead yearly conferences at the university to report on the findings.[156] Over the next thirteen years as a professor at Atlanta University, he taught, wrote, and began to receive more recognition for his ideas. At the same time, he found life in segregated Atlanta to be distressing. Although he stayed on campus to avoid personal mistreatment, it was not hard to see that, far from disappearing, segregation, discrimination, and violence had gotten worse.

In the face of these disheartening trends, Du Bois began to question the value of his research. During the years at Atlanta, as he aged from twenty-nine to forty-two, he worked hard, conducted high-quality research, and grew more accepting of others.[157] Less elitist than in his younger years and more understanding of others who were less gifted and diligent, he made new friends and developed strong relationships with the African American community in Atlanta. What discouraged him was the fact that the white world had no interest in learning the truth about African Americans. It was idealistic, he realized, to expect that scientific facts alone would persuade white leaders and the public to adopt social reforms and change behaviors.[158]

In the face of resistance to change in race relations, Du Bois felt that he could no longer be "a calm, cool, and detached social scientist."[159] He had seen firsthand the terrible odds African Americans faced in trying to improve their lives.[160] He had seen the use of fraud and intimidation to prevent African Americans from voting, the practices of the Jim Crow South in action, and the existence of a caste system that violated all democratic norms. One nearby event, the Atlanta race riot of 1906, was deeply upsetting. In response to allegations that Black men had assaulted white women, up to ten thousand whites roamed through the city in mobs hunting for African Americas. They killed dozens, injured many more, and destroyed homes and businesses.

Du Bois became involved with a group of African American leaders who advocated for a new, more militant approach to gaining rights for African Americans. In 1909, he cofounded the

National Association for the Advancement of Colored People, now known as the NAACP. The new organization demanded equal opportunity to vote, attend schools, and get jobs. It faced a daunting, near impossible mission but would do much to end segregation in decades to come. Du Bois resigned from Atlanta University in 1910, moved to New York City, and became director of publications and research of the new organization and edited its magazine.[161] He continued writing but did so outside of the academic world. In good part owing to his activities while at the NAACP, Du Bois became "the premier architect of the civil rights movement in the United States."[162]

He continued his writings and political activism until his death in 1963 at age ninety-five. He would write sixteen books on a wide variety of topics.[163] One of these, *The Souls of Black Folk* (1903), has been called "possibly the most important book ever penned by a black American."[164] In that work, Du Bois presciently noted that "the problem of the Twentieth Century is the problem of the color line."[165] As he grew older, after years and decades of struggle for racial equality, Du Bois became more radical in his political views. Still later in life, he adopted a more internationalist outlook and joined in the Pan-African movement against colonial control of people of color. He became a citizen of Ghana in 1963 and died in that country.[166]

Du Bois lived to see the initial progress toward racial equality brought about by the civil rights movement of the 1960s. He died on August 27, one day before Martin Luther King Jr. delivered his "I Have a Dream" speech at the 1963 March on Washington. The civil rights movement succeeded in ending formal segregation and improving the protection of the rights of African Americans. It did not end the economic and health inequalities between the races that Du Bois described so well. Philadelphia, the Seventh Ward, and the white and Black neighborhoods of the city illustrate the as-yet-unrealized goals of Du Bois and others.

A follow-up study of the Seventh Ward during the 1920s to the 1940s, three decades after Du Bois's study, "found insufficient water supply and toilet facilities, defective sanitary equipment, overcrowding, leaky roofs, plaster and paper falling off the walls, and windowless rooms."[167] Later, as African Americans felt new optimism from the civil rights movement, Philadelphia and other northern cities faced a new development. As African Americans gained better access to well-paying manufacturing jobs, the economy of the cities shifted away from manufacturing, and jobs moved overseas. The transition to finance and high-tech industries eliminated many of the working-class jobs that white immigrants had used in the past as stepping stones to upward mobility.[168] African American opportunities for similar mobility shrank.

The Seventh Ward today, more than 120 years after Du Bois published his book, has become mostly white. Like gentrifying parts of other cities, it has many young professionals, refurbished buildings, and businesses catering to affluent urbanites.[169] Most African Americans live elsewhere in the city, and their former churches, stores, and businesses are gone as well.[170] Elijah Anderson, currently a retired African American professor at the University of Pennsylvania with a distinguished record of publications on race, summarizes the discouraging lack of progress:

> Is the African-American of today, in Philadelphia or anywhere in the United States, free of the forces DuBois chronicled? Despite undeniable progress, the answer must be no. By considering the status of blacks then and now, the entrenched nature of the forces of both white racism and black victimization can be seen in even sharper relief than was visible to DuBois. DuBois's keen observations should make it clear to all that much additional effort will be needed before our society approaches real equality of opportunity or the rational benevolence envisioned by this eloquent, humane, and seminal thinker.[171]

Indeed, Du Bois predicted such an outcome if Americans failed to take race problems seriously.[172]

Social Epidemiology

If the promised benefits of reform that Du Bois sought remain in good part unfulfilled in American society, his insights into the causes of racial health disparities have become an essential part of public health. Recent research has revealed, for example, that experiences of discrimination and the resulting stress adversely affect health.[173] Residential segregation concentrates disadvantaged groups in the poorest areas of cities with low-quality housing, limited food choices, and few opportunities for physical activity.[174] And African Americans still receive poorer health care than whites.[175] A gap in life expectancy remains, with non-Hispanic whites living 5.9 years longer on average than non-Hispanic African Americans in 2020.[176] Most recently, the COVID-19 pandemic has widened the gap. Du Bois was well ahead of his time in linking health problems to the disadvantaged social conditions of African Americans.

The Philadelphia Negro was an early exemplar of a social epidemiological study.[177] Others at the time had examined the relationship between poverty and disease in Europe, but the application of a social perspective to the race-based distribution of disease and death was an innovation. Social epidemiology today follows the path forged by Du Bois in giving special attention to multiple forms of discrimination as causes of disease, much as Edwin Chadwick, John Snow, and Harvey Wiley gave special attention to poor sanitation, water contamination, and food adulteration as causes of disease.

Social epidemiology likewise follows Du Bois in rejecting altogether the treatment of race as a biological category. Race has importance as a socially created and maintained system of domination and a justification for that domination.[178] Resulting inequalities, inequities, or disparities are viewed as unfair and remediable rather than inevitable.[179] The term "structural racism" has emerged most recently to encompass "the macrolevel systems, social forces, institutions, ideologies, and processes that interact with one another to generate and reinforce inequities among racial and ethnic groups."[180] The work of public health depends on understanding these underlying large-scale forces and the central role of racial inequality in health.[181] Although the major histories of public health fail to mention Du Bois,[182] his work, like social epidemiology more generally, has a central place in understanding the sources of poor health.

6.

The Data Analyst
Richard Doll and Smoking

In 1946, a young English physician, Richard Doll, faced a difficult decision about what to do with his career. He had spent the past six years serving as a medical corpsman in World War II. He had braved bombs from the Luftwaffe when escaping across the English Channel just ahead of Nazi troops advancing through France.[1] He later provided medical care to wounded soldiers and almost died from kidney disease. After life-threatening adventures and the defeat of Germany in the war, he returned to the pedestrian civilian world to look for work as a doctor. Having finished his medical training nearly ten years before, he had limited choices.[2] Plus, the masses of soldiers returning to civilian work led to a crowded labor market.

Adding to the difficulty was the internal conflict he felt over two visions of an ideal career. On one hand, Doll had long been a social activist committed to justice and equitable treatment of poor people.[3] His attraction to socialism and communism emerged while still a teenager and strengthened during medical school. Holding radical political views and joining social protests during

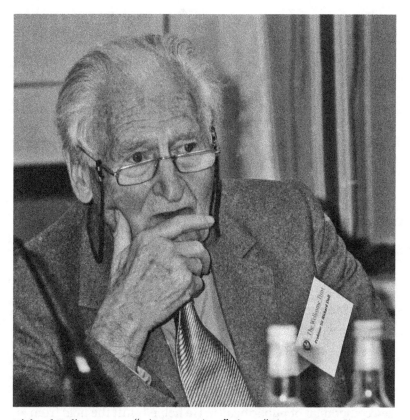

Richard Doll, 1999, at a "witness seminar" about "The MRC [Medical Research Council] Epidemiology Unit (South Wales)." *Source:* Wikimedia Commons, from the History of Modern Biomedicine Research Group. Creative Commons CC BY-SA 4.0.

the depression of the 1930s set him apart from most in the medical profession. His strong political opposition to fascism led him to serve in the armed forces during World War II. After the war, Doll desired a career that would help people and uphold his political and social commitments.

On the other hand, Doll had always been attracted to the largely solitary work of mathematics. Scientific research fit his nature better than did clinical medicine.[4] He had an impressive and even intimidating personality but one that most people viewed as detached. His strong commitment to helping people went beyond the individual lives of those he knew.[5] He felt most comfortable with the scientific pursuit of reliable data and accurate mathematical analysis.

Not many careers could meld the detached objectivity of a mathematician with a passionate commitment to social justice. Through happenstance, Doll found—and in some ways created—a career that combined both ambitions. He used scientific methods and statistical analysis for a worthy social goal: to prove the harm of tobacco use for health and thereby save lives through smoking prevention. By demonstrating beyond a reasonable doubt that cigarette smoking caused a variety of cancers, vascular diseases, respiratory diseases, and other illnesses, he advanced the goals of public health. Physicians, government officials, politicians, lawyers, anti-tobacco advocates, and citizen activists throughout the world would use Doll's findings to make healthy behavior the norm rather than the exception.

With his application of careful data analysis to health problems, Doll helped establish the legitimacy of epidemiology as a key component of public health. He helped shift the field from an exclusive focus on infectious diseases to a focus on cancer, heart disease, respiratory disease, and other chronic conditions that had come to predominate in modern societies. Epidemiology studies the incidence, distribution, and causes of disease in populations to prevent and control health problems. It is a data-driven field that focuses on populations rather than individuals and relies heavily on statistical analysis rather than clinical judgment or laboratory research. Doll's research on smoking and more generally on the environmental causes of cancer made him "the world's preeminent cancer epidemiologist" and "offered a framework for epidemiologic research that has guided investigators around the world."[6]

Many have contributed to our understanding of the harm of to-bacco use, but Doll stands out for his initial groundbreaking re-search and for another fifty-five years of continued research that silenced critics and encouraged anti-tobacco efforts. He led a rev-olution in medicine by demonstrating the value of medical sta-tistics. As portrayed in the *British Medical Journal*, he became "perhaps Britain's most eminent doctor."[7] He lived to age ninety-two, enjoyed an "extraordinarily productive life," and saw univer-sal acceptance of his work.[8]

Few need convincing today of the importance to public health of demonstrating the harm of tobacco use and reducing its world-wide prevalence. In the late 1940s, about the time Doll began his research, an astounding 80 percent of men in Britain smoked. Not surprisingly, lung cancer rates in the country were among the highest in the world.[9] Today, about 17 percent of men and women in the United Kingdom smoke daily.[10] In the United States, 55 percent of men and 25 percent of women smoked regularly in 1955.[11] By 2020, the figures had fallen to 14 percent for men and, after rising to a peak of 34 percent, to 11 percent among women.[12] The number of cigarettes consumed per person rose from 54 per year in 1900 to 4,345 at the peak in 1963 and then dropped to 1,078 in 2015.[13]

Smoking remains "the leading cause of preventable disease, disability, and death in the United States."[14] It is discouraging that about 12 percent of adults continue to smoke despite the well-known harm of tobacco and the public health efforts to eliminate the habit. But in historical perspective, the progress made through the work of Richard Doll, other researchers, a vigorous anti-tobacco movement, legal challenges to the tobacco industry, and government action has been impressive. Doll stopped smoking at age thirty-seven, and, along with extending his own life, "his work helped prevent millions of other premature deaths."[15] He managed to enjoy the scientific and mathematical work he loved while still holding to the social justice ideal of distributing the benefits of medical science to all. The blending of the two visions characterizes the field of public health today.

Surprising Unawareness about the Harm of Tobacco Use

In 1948, a medical student named Ernst Wynder observed an autopsy at Bellevue Hospital in New York City. Wynder had come to the United States only ten years earlier. He was born in Germany in 1922 to Jewish parents who fled the country to escape Nazi persecution.[16] The move to the United States must have been difficult for him, but Wynder thrived. He attended New York University, graduated with a bachelor's degree in 1943, and served in US army intelligence units during World War II.[17] In 1947, he began medical school at Washington University in St. Louis, Missouri. A summer internship at New York University brought him to an autopsy that day. The diagnosis was that the man had died of lung cancer. Although a new student and naive about the causes of cancer, Wynder asked a question that aroused his curiosity: Was the man a smoker?[18] No one there knew. The medical records listed nothing on smoking or nonsmoking—none of the physicians had seen fit to include such information. Only after asking the deceased's wife did he find out that the man had smoked two packs a day for years.[19]

At the time, Wynder would have thought little about the harm of smoking as it related to contracting lung cancer or any other disease. Few studies had investigated the link. His supervisors had not mentioned it, and it did not come up from anyone else at the autopsy. He had no solid reason to suspect a relationship. Even so, common sense might have suggested that it was not healthy to inhale smoke from burning tobacco into the throat and down to the lungs where chemicals could attach to the lining and be absorbed into the blood. Cigarettes had been called "coffin nails" decades earlier, and prohibitionist groups advocated, often successfully, for outlawing cigarettes. By 1948, however, the medical profession had largely dismissed worries about tobacco use.

Still curious, Wynder decided to investigate the possible link. One case established nothing, but perhaps investigation would reveal more. Wynder was not one to let things go. He had "brains, energy, and ambition," but the high opinion he had of himself alienated other students: "his angular face often bore a world-weary, even distasteful expression that looked as if he had just detected an unpleasant aroma."[20] Without any support or encouragement, he received permission to interview lung cancer patients at Bellevue Hospital about their disease, background, jobs, and smoking habits.[21] To establish something of a control group, he also interviewed patients with other diseases. After checking the first twenty cases, he could see a strong association between cigarette smoking and lung cancer.[22]

Richard Doll began to study smoking and lung cancer at about the same time as Wynder. He had been smoking since age seventeen.[23] Even during medical school, he gave little thought to the potential harm to his health. He certainly had not learned of the connection during his medical training and had no long-standing interest in the topic. The medical community in Britain showed the same unawareness about the danger of smoking as did that in the United States.

Nevertheless, by the late 1940s, Doll, Wynder, and most physicians very likely knew of the disconcerting acceleration of lung cancer deaths over the previous twenty years. In the United States, the male age-adjusted lung cancer death rate in 1930 of 4.3 per million people had risen to 22.6 per million people by 1948.[24] In England and Wales, the male rate rose by 10 percent per year from 1911 to 1955.[25] For the first time, lung cancer deaths exceeded tuberculosis deaths.[26] Cigarette consumption had been rising over the same time span. Smoking caused harm only after many years and decades of use rather than immediately, but one would think it easy to notice the coinciding trends of cigarette use and lung cancer and at least posit a hypothesis about smoking and premature death. Indeed, the history of tobacco use in England and the United States gave plenty of reasons for concern.

The Attractions and Dangers of Tobacco Use

Concerns about the detriments of tobacco use date back five hundred years, since the time of its importation to Europe. The tobacco plant, native to the Americas and first cultivated around 5000 BCE in present-day Peru and Ecuador, was found by users to induce a mildly pleasurable experience when dried, chopped, inserted into a pipe, and smoked. Native Americans used it in religious ceremonies, as a medicine, and to help prepare for battle.[27] As is well known, Christopher Columbus received a gift of tobacco leaves that he and his sailors brought back to Europe. In the next century, many there proclaimed the wonderous properties of the plant. Jean Nicot from France promoted the product so enthusiastically that the crucial chemical of tobacco, nicotine, was named after him. In England, Sir Walter Raleigh popularized smoking tobacco in a pipe and started something of a craze. But many warned of tobacco's dangers. Most famously, King James I of England published an anti-tobacco pamphlet in 1604 that called the custom "loathsome to the eye, hateful to the nose, harmful to the brain, dangerous to the lungs."[28]

Early warnings about the potential harm of tobacco continued. In the 1790s, Benjamin Rush, a physician and one of the signers of the Declaration of Independence, warned of the dangers of smoking, and a German physician, Samuel Thomas von Sömmerring, noticed that pipe smokers were developing cancer of the lip.[29] There was no systematic evidence, such as John Snow developed to link cholera with impure drinking water, but the public saw a connection. *Harper's Weekly*, a widely circulated newspaper, published an article in 1867 on the dangers of tobacco use as related to cancer, heart disease, and lung cancer.[30] A cartoon around the same time depicted a well-dressed man surrounded by smoke and captioned "Swell struggles with the Cig'rette Poisoner." The addictive nature of tobacco was well recognized, as illustrated in newspaper and magazine ads that promised to cure the addiction.

Worries about tobacco intensified with the production and sale of a relatively new product—manufactured cigarettes. For much of the nineteenth century, most people avoided the common forms of tobacco, mainly cigars, chew, loose tobacco, and pipe tobacco. Inhalation of pipe and cigar smoke was unpleasant, rolling cigarettes by hand was tedious, and the spit from tobacco chew was unsanitary. The invention in 1880 of a cigarette-rolling machine allowed for mass production of an innovative product. It made it possible to efficiently manufacture cigarettes in a standardized form and sell them at a low price. The new cigarettes were stylish, easy to carry and use, and most important, able to efficiently deliver nicotine to the lungs. Many soldiers during World War I (and later during World War II) learned to smoke cigarettes to deal with boredom and fear, but others adopted the habit to keep up with the new fashion.

Cigarettes addicted users much more readily than pipes, cigars, or chew—a chief objection among the anti-tobacco movements that emerged in the late 1880s. Like the temperance movement, the anti-tobacco movement found its base in rural areas and small cities, particularly among Protestant religious groups. If primarily moral in nature, opposition to cigarettes nonetheless emphasized the health dangers of smoking. Slang terms such as "the little white slaver" (used by Henry Ford in 1914) highlighted the addictiveness and "coffin nails" (used by the head of the

Anti-Cigarette League in the early 1900s) highlighted the threat to health.[31] The movement enjoyed some success with this two-pronged critique of cigarettes. Fifteen states prohibited the sale of tobacco between 1890 and 1930.[32] Like the prohibition of alcohol, however, the prohibition of tobacco did not last. The backlash against the temperance movement, the widespread violation of the anti-tobacco laws, and the spread of smoking among soldiers in World War I led states to rescind their laws by 1927.[33] The popularity of cigarettes, which by the 1920s had spread to women, seemed to push health concerns of the past into the background.

Early Studies

By the 1920s, a few researchers managed to dispute the pernicious complacency about cigarette use. Two American studies in the late 1920s noted the unusually high rates of lung cancer among heavy smokers.[34] A 1939 German study found that lung-cancer patients reported having smoked more than healthy controls, and other studies in Germany and the Netherlands during or shortly after World War II confirmed these findings.[35] In the United States, a 1938 study led by Raymond Pearl used medical records of patients available at the Johns Hopkins School of Hygiene and Public Health to study smoking. He reported that 45 percent of smokers lived to age sixty compared to 65 percent of nonsmokers.[36]

Although scattered, the evidence was there if health experts looked closely. They mostly ignored or dismissed the results. Doll later said that "the ubiquity of the habit . . . had dulled the collective sense that tobacco might be a major threat to health."[37] At the time, doctors smoked like everyone else. Some lent their names to ads claiming health benefits of smoking, and some offered patients a cigarette before an exam to reduce anxiety. Many physicians enjoyed smoking as a release from their high-stress jobs.[38] They preferred not to entertain the possibility that the habit would kill them. When Wynder, having returned from New York City to Washington University, proposed to continue his study of lung cancer and smoking, one physician puffed on his cigarette while stating with certainty that smoking did not cause lung cancer.[39] Wynder's adviser, Evarts Graham, was also skeptical but agreed to help gather national data that extended the earlier research in New York City. Neither Wynder nor Graham could foresee what influence the research would come to exert.

Even those open to new evidence thought about disease in a way that was not suited to understanding the link between smoking and lung cancer. Physicians felt most comfortable with individual patients rather than statistics and probabilities. They could point to nonsmokers who died of lung cancer and to smokers who did not die of lung cancer. The nature and causes of this type of noncommunicable disease clearly differed from those of infectious diseases. Understanding the harm of smoking required new forms of thinking about the causes of disease.

The more hardheaded methodologists pointed out flaws in the scattered evidence. Some questioned the statistics on the rise of lung cancer. The growing skills of pathologists and emerging medical interest in noncommunicable diseases likely improved the ability to detect less obvious cancers than in the past.[40] More accurate identification of lung cancer rather than the greater incidence of the disease might explain the rise. Critics also said that smoking data dependent on the recall of decade-old memories could not be trusted. Even those accepting the quality of the data identified another problem. Any association between smoking and lung cancer could be spuriously due to confounding factors. The connection of pipe smoking to lip cancer was said to be caused by the heat of the pipe stem rather than tobacco.[41] Doll originally thought that atmospheric pollution from the fumes of burning coal, the tarring of roads, and motor vehicle exhaust likely accounted for rising lung cancer.[42] Increasing atmospheric pollution coincided with both rising lung cancer and rising cigarette use. Other irritative factors such as the gassing of men during World War I were proposed to account for rising lung cancer.[43] *JAMA*, the *Journal of the American Medical Association*, summarized the consensus in 1948 that the preponderance of evidence did not indicate that tobacco was a public health problem.[44]

Tobacco companies did all they could to dismiss or hide any health concerns about cigarette smoking. They fully succeeded, largely through advertising, as smoking cigarettes became ever more popular. After World War I, when many soldiers had started to smoke, cigarette advertisements associated the habit with patriotism. Sports stars and celebrities who gave testimonials on the pleasures of smoking managed to associate cigarettes with physical fitness, strength, and glamour.[45] To double the size of the potential market, tobacco companies began to target women in the 1920s. Images of cigarettes as stylish rather than disreputable appealed to a new generation of women. Lucky Strike cigarettes claimed that physicians favored their brand because it soothed the nerves, controlled eating, reduced weight, and encouraged physical fitness.[46] The positive publicity, attraction to cigarettes, and dependence on nicotine led the public and the medical community to dismiss concerns about the injuries to health.

A Chance Occurrence

Only by chance did Richard Doll become the world's most famous epidemiologist. Born in 1912 to a physician father and concert pianist mother,[47] he enjoyed a pleasant, middle-class upbringing.[48] He attended an elite secondary school in London, where he excelled in mathematics and made plans to study it in college. When his exam results did not qualify him for a scholarship at

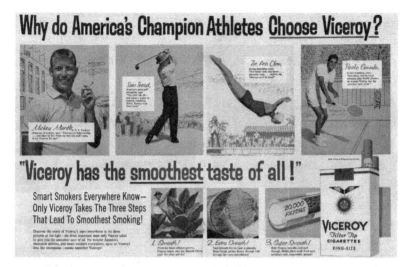

A 1957 cigarette advertisement for Viceroy cigarettes, featuring Mickey Mantle, Sam Snead, Zoe Ann Olsen, and Pancho Gonzales. *Source*: Wikimedia Commons, from the Stanford School of Medicine.

Cambridge, he decided instead to study medicine at St. Thomas Hospital in London.[49] Although he planned to become a brain surgeon, the entrance of England into war against Germany interrupted his plans. By the time Doll could return to his studies, he had no desire to go through the extensive additional training needed for neurology and surgery.[50]

Social activism became part of Doll's life while attending medical school in London from 1931 to 1937. He had already turned away from religion toward pacifism and socialism and joined the Young Communist League while a teen.[51] Medical school, where he saw firsthand the damage done to unemployed workers and others living in poverty during the Depression, strengthened his leftist views.[52] The patients he visited in the city slums lived in shockingly unhealthy conditions and received substandard health care, which differed markedly from that available to affluent sick people. The lack of understanding that most physicians had of poor people's circumstances led them to prescribe unaffordable drugs and recommend unrealistic therapies.[53] He came to believe that lasting improvement for the health of people in economic distress required broad social change more than individual medical treatment. Toward that end, he organized a socialist society at the medical school, joined the Communist Party, and participated in protests and marches.[54] Showing his commitment to communism, Doll traveled to the Soviet Union at age twenty-one.[55] He would reject communism many years later but not the goal of improving public health through social action.

Everything changed in 1939. Having recognized the danger of Nazi Germany and the threat of fascism, Doll had volunteered the previous year for the Army Medical Corps Reserve. When war broke out, he was called up immediately for active duty.[56] While serving in France, "he treated and helped evacuate many wounded through the chaotic retreat to Dunkirk, despite sustained shelling and air attack, taking charge when other officers were lost, and leading men to safety."[57] He then went to Egypt in 1941 as a medical officer and later served on a hospital ship that supported the invasion of Italy by the Allies. Only in 1944, after he developed tuberculosis of the kidney and had a kidney removed, did he leave the armed forces.[58] Later in life, Doll noted with irony that, as one of the few survivors of Dunkirk, his war experiences attracted more media attention than his scientific research.[59]

While at a meeting of communist doctors in the early 1930s, Doll met his wife-to-be, Joan Mary Faulkner, who was married at the time.[60] They shared a commitment to social activism and radical reform. Doll proposed to her in 1945 at the end of the war, and after she finalized her divorce, the two married in 1949.[61] Joan had a son from her previous marriage but was unable to have more children. When the couple tried to adopt, agencies rejected them as suitable parents because of their avowed atheism. They set up their own humanist adoption agency and adopted two children, Nicholas in 1954 and Catherine in 1956.[62] Joan also worked in the field of medical research, and together they formed an influential partnership.[63] By all accounts, the couple loved each other deeply.[64]

After the war, Doll found few promising opportunities to practice medicine or continue advanced medical studies.[65] It was not an easy time to obtain work, especially for someone known to medical colleagues for his communist beliefs.[66] He returned briefly to St. Thomas Hospital, where he had received his medical training, but disliked the work and decided to look for a research job.[67] He ended up taking a position as a research assistant with a gastroenterologist doing a study of occupation and peptic ulcers.[68] The work involved epidemiology, a new field for Doll but one requiring the use of math and statistics and careful persistence in gathering data. He excelled at the tasks.

Doll's career took the course it would follow for the rest of his life with a class on medical statistics taught by A. Bradford Hill.[69] Hill learned of Doll's work on peptic ulcers and found it so impressive that he offered his former student a position in 1948 at the Statistical Research Unit of the Medical Research Council.[70] Hill directed the unit, which had been investigating the environmental causes of disease. The job not only suited Doll's mathematical talents but also his social conscience. Epidemiological studies were well suited for understanding large-scale public health problems and developing strategies of social change to address the problems.

At the time, Hill had been asked to lead a study on smoking and lung cancer. The chief medical officer of the General Register Office held the rare view that increasing lung cancer deaths involved something more than improved diagnoses.[71] Hill put Doll on the project but likely did not yet realize how valuable the new colleague would become. Given the flaws of existing studies, reading the literature did not convince Doll to change his dismissive views on the topic. He certainly had no grand plans to improve public health by preventing tobacco use. In fact, he smoked both a pipe and cigarettes at the time and admitted that he was not antagonistic to tobacco when he started the study.[72] Anti-tobacco views would come later. For the time being, he simply saw an interesting epidemiological problem that needed careful study.

Doll presented an impressive if daunting figure. He was elegant, articulate, well-mannered, and handsomely dressed.[73] Acquaintances described him as charming and approachable and as "witty, winning, every bit the gentleman."[74] At the same time, he was self-confident in a way that could come across as arrogant and intimidating. He worked hard, was highly knowledgeable, and expressed his opinions with self-assurance. He spoke and wrote clearly, carefully, and factually, and expected the same from others.[75] Because of his commitment to his studies and workaholic personality, he often seemed detached and unemotional.[76] That made him both respected and feared. In the words of an admirer, he was committed to "help both individuals and causes where he saw an injustice, but otherwise showed little interest in other people's personal lives."[77] He was too busy with his work. He said that, outside of work, his home was his major interest and source of enjoyment and that he enjoyed literature, the theater, and traveling. But even then he mentioned a worklike commitment to establishing a new college in Oxford.[78] He "found good epidemiology beautiful and satisfying, considering himself to have been extraordinarily lucky professionally."[79] Through good fortune plus hard work and considerable talent, Doll at age thirty-seven "stood on the threshold of making one of the defining medical discoveries of the 20th century."[80]

The Case-Control Study

Converging Findings

Doll and Hill set to work on their new project. As Hill had warned, few in the medical profession at the time took kindly to careful statistical analysis.[81] That would change through use of a strategy—the case-control design—that, although not altogether new, had not yet been fully exploited. It would eventually become a mainstay of epidemiological research. As applied by Doll and Hill, the logic of the design was straightforward: Identify two groups of hospital patients, one with lung cancer and one with different diseases. The two groups should be located in the same hospitals and be similar in age, sex, residence, and social class. Then the researchers would work backward to find out how the two groups differed in terms of past behaviors, exposures, physical characteristics, and other factors that might be associated with the disease. The retrospective approach began with the outcome and traced back to find likely causes.

Step one for Doll and Hill involved creating a detailed questionnaire on smoking. Questions covered one's status as a current smoker, former smoker, or never smoker. Current and former smokers were asked about the age of starting and former smokers about the age when they stopped. Other smoking details included the type of tobacco (pipe, cigars, cigarettes), the amount normally smoked, and the extent of inhaling. The design of such questions was harder than it sounds. Smoking habits change, and irregular, occasional, and experimental smokers fit poorly into broad categories. For example, one woman in the study said she smoked one cigarette a year after Christmas dinner, and one man said he tried smoking a few cigarettes when young.[82] Doll and Hill thought these cases did not qualify as smokers. They came up with a precise definition of a smoker that made enough sense to be widely adopted by other studies: a person who smoked at least one cigarette a day for a year. With answers to the questions, the researchers could compare never smokers to former and current smokers as well as compare light, medium, and heavy smokers.

Step two involved selection of the sample to interview. Twenty cooperating hospitals agreed to notify all patients with carcinoma of the lung, stomach, colon, or rectum of the study. Four women, quaintly called "almoners" by Doll and Hill, were hired to visit these patients and interview them using the detailed questionnaire constructed for the study.[83] But that was not enough. For each cancer patient the women interviewed, they needed to find another patient at the same hospital who was of the same gender and age group but did not have cancer. Being in the same hospital would mean that both the cancerous and noncancerous patients likely came from the same part of town and had been exposed to much the same air pollution. Being the same gender and age meant that differences between the patients in the two groups would not result from physical characteristics. The two sets of patients would thus be similar enough to isolate the impact of smoking.

Data obtained from 1,732 patients with cancer and the 743 general medical and surgical patients allowed for reliable comparisons.[84] The results demonstrated that lung cancer patients were more likely to be smokers than other patients. Doll found the results so convincing that he stopped smoking cigarettes.[85] But Doll and Hill were cautious in their scientific conclusions. They knew the results would be unpopular and wanted to check and eliminate alternative explanations. On the recommendation of a colleague, they decided to strengthen their case by gathering more data outside of London.[86] In the meantime, Ernst Wynder and Evarts Graham had finished their case-control study of American patients. When Doll and Hill saw the published article in early 1950, they decided to publish their results right away.

The year 1950 marks the starting point of the ongoing battle to eliminate the use of tobacco and cigarettes. That year saw the publication of five studies, each demonstrating more reliably than anything previously written that cigarette smoking was associated with lung cancer. Most widely read were the articles by Wynder and Graham in the *Journal of the American Medical Association* and by Doll and Hill in the *British Medical Journal*.[87] These two studies used large samples and carefully implemented case-control designs. The other three articles, although less famous and influential, reinforced the findings. The articles converged on the harm of tobacco in a way that challenged the widespread thinking about smoking. They also demonstrated the value of an epidemiological approach to understanding the sources of disease. Publication of the articles marked the end of the age of innocence about smoking.[88]

A review of the results of Doll and Hill illustrates the kind of evidence first used to make the case against tobacco.[89] Start with male patients having lung carcinoma. Nearly all these men, 99.7 percent, smoked. For the other patients, however, smokers were less common—95.8 percent. Smoking was prevalent in both groups, but the gap between the two groups exceeded what would be expected by chance. The numbers for women, who were less likely to smoke, revealed a larger gap. Among lung cancer patients, 68.3 percent were smokers versus 46.7 percent among the other patients. The 21.6 percent difference indicated a strong relationship between smoking and lung cancer. The extent of exposure to the potential harm from smoking further strengthened the findings. Compare heavy smokers with light smokers. The heavy smokers were more likely than light smokers to come from the group of lung cancer patients. Similarly, cigarette smokers compared to pipe smokers were more vulnerable to lung cancer, and those who started earlier and smoked for more years were more vulnerable than those who smoked for shorter periods. Doll and Hill summarized, "It must be concluded that there is a real association between carcinoma of the lung and smoking."[90] In fact, they believed that the association was causal. They added, "Nor can we ourselves envisage any common cause likely to lead to both the development of the habit and to the development of the disease 20 to 50 years later."[91]

The study by Ernst Wynder and Evarts Graham in the United States produced results quite similar to those of Doll and Hill. Together, the two studies strengthened the reliability of the findings. Wynder and Graham examined 605 cases of proven bronchiogenic carcinoma in hospitals across the United States.[92] The study also examined a group of 780 control patients in hospitals without the disease. The results clearly demonstrated a difference. The general population of male patients had 14.6 percent nonsmokers, while the male lung cancer patients had only 1.3 percent nonsmokers. There were 54.7 percent heavy smokers in the general population of male patients compared to 86.4 percent among male lung cancer patients. The authors concluded in cautious but clear language that "the temptation is strong to incriminate excessive smoking, and in particular cigarette smoking, over a long period as at least one important factor in the striking increase in branchiogenic carcinoma."[93]

Neither of the two articles made explicit recommendations for stopping the rise in smoking-related cancers. Knowing of the unpopularity of such a recommendation, the authors concentrated on presenting a scientifically thorough analysis of the association. At the time, Doll said that he did not want to become emotionally attached to his findings or campaign publicly for them.[94] But most anyone could see the implications. Rather than treating the disease after its occurrence, public health measures would be better deployed to focus on people's behavior, to prevent them from smoking in the first place.

Government officials and the tobacco industry responded with caution and hostility, respectively.[95] The bureaucrats had little to say about the methods but wanted to avoid making a startling recommendation about tobacco or publicly campaigning against smoking. In Doll's view, "advisors to the government were pathologically scared of causing cancer phobia by undertaking any publicity about cancer, even to the extent of opposing education about the need for early diagnosis. Within government there was anxiety about the effects of reduced sales on tax income and there was certainly a desire to work with the industry rather than against it."[96] The government wanted consensus from scientists and media publicity about the harm of tobacco before taking a stand. Even then, as Doll notes, the reliance of the government on taxes from tobacco companies inhibited their action. In England, about 14 percent of the government's revenue came from tobacco.[97]

Tobacco companies certainly recognized the threat that the research presented to their business. The massive sales of cigarettes and generous profits lent them a good deal of economic and political power. One strategy was to lobby the government to prevent any public anti-tobacco pronouncements. Another was to hire experts to dispute the findings and criticize the limitations of the case-control studies. The critics could exploit the general resistance in the medical community to epidemiological studies. Only after overcoming this resistance could public health leaders take full advantage of the case-control findings.

Statisticians Debate Causality

It is easy to understand the motivations of government officials and tobacco executives who wanted to protect their interests. And, not surprisingly, a detailed article filled with statistics and published in a medical journal had little influence on the general public. However, the negative reaction to the findings from physicians, scientists, and cancer researchers surprised Doll.[98] Many may have simply not wanted to confront the fact that a habit they enjoyed might kill them—it would be easier to deny the findings than to quit smoking. At the same time, some researchers had sincere concerns about the validity of observational findings such as Doll and Hill presented.

Many viewed epidemiology and its reliance on statistical analysis as a soft science, one unable to identify the real causes of disease.[99] They wanted to see clinical and experimental data. One could easily observe that, for example, patients recovered from sickness following a shot of penicillin or that a new drug or medical procedure worked better than a placebo when a treatment group and a control group were randomly assigned and statistically identical except for the treatment. These kinds of studies, unlike epidemiological studies, could identify the causes of disease with some certainty. Such experiments obviously did not work for understanding the harm of smoking for humans. The effects occurred only after a lag of decades, and experimenters could not randomly assign people to start or not start smoking. Doll, Hill, Wynder, Graham, and the few other researchers struggling "to demonstrate through science that smoking caused human cancer often felt alone."[100]

The larger question concerned the usual standard of proof of causality in medical science: Did the standard used for the study of infectious diseases apply to the study of diseases such as cancers? A key postulate laid out by the German microbiologist Robert Koch in the late 1800s had guided medical science. It stated that, to establish a causal relationship, the source of a disease should be found in abundance among those with the disease but not among those without the disease. For example, *Vibrio cholerae* bacteria were found in cholera victims but not in others. Epidemiological research, in contrast, dealt with probabilities, not certainties. Doll and Hill demonstrated that the probability of getting lung cancer was significantly higher for smokers than nonsmokers, but exceptions were common. Many other causes must be involved to explain the exceptions. Understanding one specific source of a disease like cancer, which results from multiple factors rather than from a single infectious agent, required new forms of medical research and new understandings of causality. It would require "a fundamental shift in scientific thinking."[101]

Many eminent statisticians and medical researchers were not ready to make such a change. The most famous, Sir Ronald Fisher, is widely considered today as one of the most important twentieth-century figures in statistical science. Fisher and others pointed out that without a true experiment, the association between smoking and lung cancer could have resulted from any number of common causes. A key principle of any introductory statistics course is that correlation does not equal causation. Applied to the smoking study, critics pointed to other causes known to affect lung cancer, such as air pollution and industrial fumes, that affected smokers more than nonsmokers. In their view, the other causes made it difficult if not impossible to isolate the effects of smoking.[102] Fisher further argued that genetic differences made smoking especially attractive to people who were prone to lung cancer and could account for the case-control results.[103] In short, without experimental evidence, the association of smoking and lung cancer could be spurious. Unfortunately, Fisher presented his criticisms with a good deal of contempt and disagreeableness that made the debate particularly heated.[104]

Doll and Hill had addressed some of these concerns.[105] The same association between smoking and lung cancer appeared among city residents exposed to auto exhaust as among residents living outside of cities who enjoyed fresher air. The same association appeared among laborers exposed to factory fumes as among white-collar workers spending time in offices. How could auto exhaust or factory fumes explain the presence of lung cancer in smokers living in places with fresh air and in people working in offices? The genetic explanation offered by Fisher also made little sense to Doll and Hill. Although they could not disprove the explanation with the data they had, they knew that the association between smoking and lung cancer also showed up in different countries and groups with different genetic backgrounds. The preponderance of the evidence favored the hypothesis that smoking caused lung cancer.

Doll and Hill believed that the medical field needed a new understanding of causality that recognized the multiple sources of many diseases. For lung cancer and other chronic diseases, smoking was neither a necessary nor sufficient cause, but it was an important cause.[106] Some nonsmokers got lung cancer, but the risk was lower than for smokers, and many smokers avoided lung cancer but much less often than nonsmokers. Although difficult for many to accept at first, heightened risk, when demonstrated by strong evidence, can imply causality.[107] Critics sought to find *the* cause rather than *a* cause of diseases that have many causes.[108]

Based on the smoking studies, Bradford Hill laid out nine criteria for establishing causality that applied to chronic diseases as well as to infectious diseases.[109] For example, there should be a strong relationship between the presence of the cause and the disease, and there should be a strong dose-response relationship in which greater exposure to the cause leads to greater presence of the disease. The disease should emerge with an appropriate interval after exposure. There should be consistency of results across studies. There should be a plausible biological mechanism behind the observed relationship. Smoking met these criteria. Hill wrote, "None of my nine viewpoints can bring indisputable evidence for or against the cause-and-effect hypothesis and none can be required as a sine qua non [essential condition]. What they can do, with greater or less strength, is to help us make up our minds on the fundamental question—is there any other way of explaining the set of facts before us."[110]

In Doll's view, the evidence from the case-control studies offered proof beyond a reasonable doubt of the harm of smoking, much the same standard used in a court of law.[111] However, something more was needed to persuade skeptics of the causal impact of smoking and produce a scientific consensus. The evidence needed to go beyond the retrospective case-control studies. Wynder began nonepidemiological research with a study of the occurrence of skin cancer after painting tobacco tar on lab animals. Doll and Hill continued their epidemiological work but now focused on a prospective study. The study would continue for fifty years and make Doll the person most identified with epidemiological research on smoking.

The Doctors Study

A prospective study first interviews a sample about smoking before the disease occurs and then follows both smokers and non-smokers to measure the future emergence of disease. The design minimizes the dependence on the possibly faulty memories of subjects about their past smoking. It also avoids a sample of possibly unrepresentative lung cancer patients in hospitals. But it requires preselecting a sample to be followed. Bradford Hill came up with the idea to study doctors.[112] A sample of doctors had several advantages over other social or occupational groups. They would be easy to locate and follow because of their medical practices, would provide accurate data because of their scientific training, and would want to participate in the project because of their interest in the medical findings.[113] If the doctors saw from the results that they were dying prematurely from smoking, they would change their behavior and encourage patients to do the same.

Doll and Hill began the study in 1951 with a survey of more than forty thousand British physicians.[114] The British Medical Association helped with a letter asking its members to participate in the study.[115] The survey included the usual set of detailed questions on current and past smoking. Unlike the case-control study, in which nearly all the male patients were smokers, the doctors varied more in their use of tobacco. For men ages thirty-five and older, 13 percent had never smoked, 35 percent were light smokers, 31 percent were moderate smokers, and 21 percent were heavy smokers.[116]

The next step used government records to obtain data on the deaths of the doctors. The researchers matched the names and identifying information from the survey of doctors to death certificates and recorded the cause of death. Over a short period of twenty-nine months, they found thirty-six deaths from lung cancer.[117] The article Doll and Hill published on the results in 1954 demonstrated that the risk of death from lung cancer rose steadily with exposure to smoking. The figures from the prospective doctors study closely matched those from the retrospective case-control study,[118] a result that brought Doll and Hill a good deal of satisfaction and vindication. Along with confirming earlier findings about the harm of tobacco for lung cancer, the study discovered something new and unexpected. Smoking was associated with many other diseases. It proved even more harmful than initially suggested by the case-control results.

In the United States, another prospective study confirmed the most recent findings of Doll and Hill. Two scientists working for the American Cancer Society, E. Cuyler Hammond and Daniel Horn, decided to check the findings of the recent case-control studies. Hammond said that they expected to disprove the claims of Wynder and Graham and Doll and Hill.[119] With help from volunteers of the American Cancer Society, they recruited nearly 188,000 men to participate in the study.[120] After obtaining detailed survey information on smoking from the sample, the researchers, again with the help of volunteers, obtained death certificate information on those who died over the next twenty months. Hammond and Horn concluded from the data that "men with a history of regular cigarette smoking have a considerably higher death rate than men who have never smoked or men who have smoked only cigars or pipes."[121] Complementing the doctor's study, this independent study done in a different country with a different sample confirmed the harm of tobacco. On seeing the results, Hammond and Horn, both heavy smokers, switched to pipes.[122]

As additional studies accumulated, the epidemiological findings steadily convinced experts of the causal impact of smoking. By 1960, the debate had largely ended, with only a few dissidents left who disputed the evidence.[123] With the evidence clearly on their side and their critics largely silenced, Doll and Hill wanted to learn more and continued their study of the doctors. A follow-up over a longer time span would include more deaths and allow for more reliable analysis of the harm of smoking. It also would have another benefit. A resurvey of the doctors could identify those who had given up smoking during the period from the first survey to the second. Comparing quitters with continuing smokers would show the potential health benefits of stopping. The still-surviving doctors responded to another survey of men in 1957–1958 and women in 1960–1961.[124]

Over the ten years of the study, from 1951 to 1961, 4,597 male doctors and 366 female doctors had died.[125] The evidence of the harm of smoking emerged more strongly than earlier. For all causes, cigarette smokers died at a rate that was 28 percent higher than nonsmokers, while pipe and cigar smokers died at a rate only 1 percent higher than nonsmokers.[126] For lung cancer specifically, the figures were more striking: the death rate of cigarette smokers was thirteen times the rate of nonsmokers, and the death rate of heavy cigarette smokers was thirty times the rate of nonsmokers.[127] In addition, those reporting in either survey that they had given up smoking had substantially fewer lung cancer deaths than continuing smokers, and the earlier smoking had stopped, the greater the reduction in lung cancer deaths.[128] Demonstrating the benefits of stopping refuted the hostile and erroneous claims of Fisher that, because the relationship between smoking and lung cancer was spuriously due to other causes, stopping smoking would bring little benefit.[129]

Doll was not done yet. With a new set of collaborators, he followed the doctors for twenty years (to 1971), then for forty years (to 1991), and finally for fifty years (to 2001). As the doctors in the study grew older, the harm of smoking became all the more indisputable. After forty years of study, Doll and his colleagues concluded "that about half of all regular cigarette smokers will eventually be killed by their habit."[130] Furthermore, those who stopped smoking before middle age "avoided almost all of the excess risk that they would otherwise have suffered," and "those who stopped smoking in middle age were subsequently at substantially less risk than those who continued to smoke."[131] After fifty years, from 1951 to 2001, 25,346 deaths occurred among the men, leaving only 5,902 who were still alive.[132] The long-term results put the harm of smoking in concrete terms: "Men born in 1900–1930 who smoked only cigarettes and continued smoking died on average about 10 years younger than lifelong nonsmokers."[133] Men who stopped at age thirty gained back all ten years of life expectancy, and men who stopped by age sixty gained back about three years of life expectancy.

The decades-long results and large sample size made it possible for Doll and colleagues to reliably establish that smoking was related to numerous cancers, chronic bronchitis, and coronary disease. Based on the doctors study and many others, the US surgeon general has summarized the current state of knowledge:

Smoking causes 87 percent of lung cancer deaths, 32 percent of coronary heart disease deaths, and 79 percent of all cases of chronic obstructive pulmonary disease (COPD) . . . [and] smoking causes diabetes mellitus, rheumatoid arthritis and immune system weakness, increased risk for tuberculosis disease and death, ectopic (tubal) pregnancy and impaired fertility, cleft lip and cleft palates in babies of women who smoke during early pregnancy, erectile dysfunction, and age-related macular degeneration.[134]

Prevention Efforts

Despite the scientific consensus that tobacco use caused lung cancer and a wide variety of other diseases, changing public policy presented a challenge. Ernst Wynder described the problem:

> From the public health point of view, the lesson to be learned is that consensus of opinion among experts is not sufficient to create action unless such consensus is translated into preventive or control measures, and this requires the experts, government, and the media and educators to act in concert. Scientists and physicians cannot be content with discoveries until their beneficial or protective outcome for the population has been fully realized. This means that the members of the scientific and medical community must become more proactive in public health matters.[135]

Epidemiological research alone did not bring about public policy changes, but prevention efforts certainly depended on strong scientific findings.

Richard Doll himself avoided public campaigning but continued to vigorously make the scientific case for the harm of tobacco use. His work provided the foundation for successful prevention efforts. After a long career at the Medical Statistics Unit, where he eventually replaced Bradford Hill as director, Doll was named in 1969 as the Regius Professor of Medicine at Oxford, the most prestigious medical position in Great Britain.[136] Appointing an epidemiologist as a professor of medicine at such a famous university brought new attention and respect to epidemiological research.[137] While increasingly occupied by administrative duties, Doll continued his research on smoking and cancer epidemiology. In 1971, he was knighted by the queen for his work and became Sir Richard.

Doll's anti-tobacco advocacy took the form of giving expert testimony, presenting invited lectures, and disputing criticisms of his scientific findings.[138] The false claims about the safety of smoking made by tobacco industry executives and researchers angered Doll and made expert testimony against tobacco companies increasingly important to his career.[139] He served as an effective witness in lawsuits. In 2002, the *Los Angeles Times* wrote about his testimony in a California suit against Philip Morris, a large and successful tobacco maker. "Dignified, affable, and decorated with honors, Doll is a tobacco lawyer's worst nightmare. He sits there with noble countenance and solid science, his virtue unimpeachable, and wins the day."[140]

Well before moving to Oxford, Doll saw his research used to justify antismoking policy changes. In 1957, the Medical Research Council concluded that there was a direct cause-and-effect relationship between smoking and lung cancer.[141] Because Hill and then Doll headed the Statistical Research Unit of the Medical Research Council, it might be expected that the organization would certify the research of its own unit. Even so, the statement had much importance—the council became the first national institution to acknowledge tobacco as a major cause of death.[142] Based in good part on the report, the Ministry of Health decided to launch an educational campaign to raise awareness on the dangers of smoking.[143]

In 1962, the Royal College of Physicians published its first report on smoking. Doing more than affirming that tobacco use harmed health, the report made policy recommendations. It called for higher taxes on cigarettes, education of the public, and restrictions on advertising, smoking in public places, and the sale of tobacco to children.[144] With the report, the government set up a cabinet committee on smoking. Although the ensuing policy changes were modest and mostly focused on education,[145] the acceptance of epidemiological findings by the medical profession signaled a critical step forward in the anti-tobacco effort.

A major change in the public perception of the harm of smoking came from a 1964 report of the US surgeon general. The 387-page report relied on approximately seven thousand articles relating to smoking and disease.[146] The review of the evidence demonstrated that smoking was a cause of lung cancer in men, a probable cause of lung cancer in women, and the most important cause of chronic bronchitis.[147] The report concluded, "Cigarette smoking is a health hazard of sufficient importance in the United States to warrant appropriate remedial action."[148]

The scientific report received unexpected publicity—and generated a good deal of anxiety among smokers. As recalled by Surgeon General Luther Terry, "The report hit the country like a bombshell. It was front-page news and a lead story on every television and radio station in the United States and many abroad. The report not only carried a strong condemnation of tobacco usage, especially cigarette smoking, but conveyed its message in such clear and concise language that it could not be misunderstood."[149] The year of its publication, 1964, marked the start of a long-term decline in cigarette consumption in the United States.[150] Congress soon responded with the Federal Cigarette Labeling and Advertising Act of 1965 and later with the Public Health Cigarette Smoking Act of 1969. The new laws took the initial and modest steps of requiring a health warning on cigarette packages and banning cigarette advertising in the broadcast media.

Prevention efforts have continued uninterrupted since then. Anti-tobacco policies include bans on smoking in airplanes, workplaces, and public buildings; increased local, state, and federal taxes on cigarettes; approval of cessation products such as nicotine patches; more severe and noticeable warnings about the hazards of cigarettes; and lawsuits against tobacco companies. The tobacco companies fought back against these changes with what can only be called a scientific disinformation campaign.[151] In 1998, however, the companies agreed to pay $246 billion over twenty-five years to the states to settle lawsuits and pay for the public costs of treating smoking-caused illnesses. Today, taxes make the purchase of cigarettes expensive enough to discourage many smokers, and smoke-free regulations limit the opportunities to smoke and the exposure of others to second-hand smoke. A graph of cigarette consumption and lung cancer deaths in the United States from 1900 through the early 2000s shows that the deaths followed the same curve as cigarette consumption, only after a lag of about two decades (see below).

The surgeon general puts these accomplishments in perspective: "The epidemic of smoking-caused disease in the twentieth

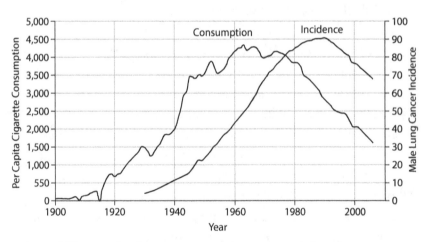

Annual US per capita cigarette consumption versus male lung cancer incidence per 100,000 men, 1900–ca. 2005. *Source*: Wikimedia Commons, adapted from Armin Kübelbeck with data from *AACR Cancer Progress Report 2012*.

century ranks among the greatest public health catastrophes of the century, while the decline of smoking consequent to tobacco control is surely one of public health's greatest successes."[152]

Epidemiology and Public Health

Over the last decades of his life, Richard Doll kept working through many adversities—a diagnosis of celiac disease, a successful operation to remove cancer from his large bowel, and the death of his beloved wife.[153] By 2005, more than twenty-five years after retiring from his position at Oxford University, he maintained an impressive schedule of traveling, lecturing, and collaborating with colleagues on new research projects.[154] He could look back with satisfaction on how central epidemiological research had become to promoting public health goals. His fame would even take a concrete form. In June 2005, the research units he founded moved into the new Richard Doll Building at Oxford University.[155] Research in the building continued Doll's work on large-scale population studies of the causes, prevention, and treatment of cancers and other chronic diseases.[156]

Soon after the building opened, Doll suffered a heart attack. He died in the hospital at age ninety-two on July 24, 2005. Even when in the hospital, he continued to work and discuss research with his colleagues.[157] A laudatory obituary illustrates the admiration he inspired:

> Days before he entered hospital, he attended the Green College summer dinner, a fine figure in a white tuxedo, charming friends young and old, and enthusing about the new building that bears his name. He drew envious glances from men, who told each other they would be happy to be half as active at 70, never mind 90, and admiring glances from women, some joking with each other that given the chance, they would leave home for him. Sir Richard Doll

used to say that he wanted to die young as old as possible. That is exactly what he did; and thanks to his life's work, millions of others have the chance of doing the same.[158]

An article in the *British Medical Journal*, "Richard Doll at 85," concisely summarized his contribution to public health and human well-being: "Two thirds of the ex-smokers [in Britain] who have survived to 85 would have died if they carried on smoking. They owe their lives to Sir Richard."[159] The same holds for ex-smokers in countries throughout the world. The lives saved came from moving "medical research out of the hospital ward and laboratory" and into society.[160] Doll resolutely believed that the science of epidemiology could directly benefit populations in ways "that could never be achieved by curative medicine alone."[161]

Many besides Doll deserve credit for improvements in health that resulted from decreased smoking. Thousands of epidemiological researchers have joined in the project to understand and prevent the harm of smoking. Doll's American colleague who shared in the initial studies of the harm of tobacco, Ernst Wynder, stands out. He died from cancer in 1999, six years before Doll. Younger than Doll when he first published his research, Wynder sadly lived only to age seventy-seven.[162] During his life, he published prolifically, mostly on cancer, and received numerous awards and honors. The field of public health benefited enormously from his contributions, much as it did from Doll's.

Doll's five hundred publications over fifty years have extended his epidemiological approach beyond tobacco. Specialized studies focused, for example, on the influence of radiation and asbestos on cancer.[163] Best known is his 1981 report with Richard Peto, *The Causes of Cancer*. The United States Congress, concerned at the time about the exposure of workers to harmful materials, commissioned the British researchers to provide estimates of the risks associated with cancer. Using data from the United States, the analysis attributed 30 percent of cancers to tobacco smoking, 35 percent to diet, 7 percent to reproductive and sexual behavior, and 5 percent occupational exposure. The study suggested that about two-thirds of all cancer cases were preventable.[164] Current research has reduced the figure on diet to closer to 16 percent, but otherwise the estimates of Doll and Peto have held up well.[165]

Doll's findings on smoking and other environmental causes of cancer changed the way physicians thought about aging and death. If most cancers were avoidable and not always the natural consequence of old age, then behavior change could extend people's lives.[166] The epidemiological approaches to public health used so successfully to describe, understand, and prevent the spread of infectious diseases could similarly be used to understand noninfectious diseases that emerged decades rather than days after exposure.

Despite the enormous success in reducing tobacco use in Britain, the United States, and most countries throughout the world, and despite the widespread understanding of the harm of smoking to health, public health efforts have much left to accomplish. In the high-income nations of western Europe and North America, a segment of the population—from roughly 11 percent in Sweden to 24 percent in Germany—continues to smoke daily.[167] The figure of 12 percent in United States falls below that of 17 percent in the United Kingdom but remains too high. Countries of eastern and southern Europe have still higher levels of smoking prevalence—33 percent in the Russian Federation and 34 percent in Greece. Also worrisome to public health advocates is the increasing concentration of smoking among less-educated and disadvantaged social groups, including many racial and ethnic minorities.[168] Special antismoking efforts are needed to target these groups.

In many less-wealthy nations, smoking prevalence remains disconcertingly high. The global smoking epidemic has been driven by large tobacco corporations that promote the use of tobacco across the world.[169] According to the World Health Organization, "The tobacco epidemic is one of the biggest public health threats the world has ever faced, killing more than 8 million people a year around the world."[170] Estimates predict that by 2030, "a shocking 1 billion people are projected to die from tobacco use this century."[171] The key components of change in high-income nations—scientific evidence, dramatic policy change, brave leadership, and control of transnational tobacco companies—are needed in the global fight to prevent tobacco-related death.[172] In combining objective science with the public good, much as Doll did for more than fifty years, epidemiology will continue to play an important role in global public health campaigns.

7.

The International Manager

D. A. Henderson and the Global Eradication of Smallpox

In 1977, Ali Maow Maalin worked as a hospital cook in Merca, Somalia, a city located on the eastern coast of Africa along the Indian Ocean. A healthy young man in his early twenties, Maalin helped with hospital vaccinations along with cooking duties. The hospital vaccinated employees and patients against smallpox, a terrible disease that in past decades had killed many in Somalia and nearby countries. Everyone presumed that Maalin, as a hospital employee who helped with vaccinations, had himself been vaccinated. In fact, he later admitted, "I was scared of being vaccinated then. It looked like the shot hurt."[1] His deception would not have mattered had not a smallpox outbreak occurred among a nomadic tribe in Somalia. Not suspecting Maalin's vulnerability, a driver asked him to help transport the smallpox victims from an encampment to the Merca hospital. Maalin agreed, traveling with the victims in a Land Cruiser for the short, five-minute trip.[2] One six-year-old girl, Habiba Nur Ali, died from the smallpox, but isolation and treatment managed to protect the others in the tribe. Officials of the World Health Organization (WHO) who

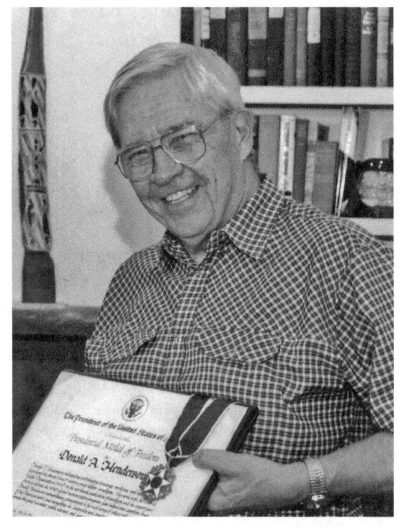

D. A. Henderson, 2002, a week after receiving the Presidential Medal of Freedom. *Source*: Wikimedia Commons.

had supervised the operation to prevent the spread of smallpox to others must have felt relieved. They believed they had contained the outbreak.

About nine days later, Maalin had a fever and headache. Doctors initially diagnosed malaria, a common disease in the area, and then chickenpox.[3] Only after being released from the hospital did it become apparent that Maalin had smallpox. The small round pustules typical of the disease covered his skin. Realizing that he had smallpox and not wanting to be isolated, Maalin fled and hid. Health officials hearing from others about Maalin's obvious smallpox markings, knew that he would spread the disease to others and destroy their efforts to protect the Somali public from the disease. They traced and vaccinated his contacts over the past days—an amazing effort of detective work. They also offered a reward for help in finding Maalin. The reward was large enough for one of Maalin's co-workers to turn him in. In the meantime, fifty-four thousand people in the area received vaccinations to prevent the disease from spreading.[4]

Despite all the trouble Maalin caused, the story ends well. Maalin recovered from smallpox, and because of the hurried vaccination of his contacts, no one else was infected. Most satisfying, Maalin turned out to be the last human on earth infected by naturally occurring smallpox. Except for samples stored in labs, the smallpox virus had, after Maalin's case in 1977, been eradicated. The scourge of smallpox, one of history's deadliest diseases, had disappeared from the human species. Maalin became semifamous for his status as the last disease carrier. After his smallpox case, he atoned for his mistakes by volunteering in the Somali program to eradicate polio. He lived to age fifty-nine, when he died of malaria.[5]

Maalin today stands as a symbol of one of humankind's greatest accomplishments. The eradication of smallpox was unprecedented, an achievement more impressive than the moon landing but much less recognized.[6] The eradication resulted from the effort of an army of workers, health officials, and organization leaders who devoted a decade to the goal. Thanks to these efforts, hundreds of millions of people in the world who would have died at young ages without the smallpox eradication program have instead lived longer and healthier lives. Estimates suggest that since 1980, 150 million to 200 million lives have been saved by smallpox vaccination.[7] Millions more who would have recovered from smallpox were spared the suffering and scarring caused by the disease.

It is hard to identify a single person most responsible for the eradication. Many credit Edward Jenner, an eighteenth-century physician who first developed and publicized a safe and effective vaccine. His discovery was a great scientific breakthrough. However, a key point of public health is that a vaccine alone does not save lives—vaccinations save lives. And vaccinations require an organizational effort to deliver the vaccine to the populations at risk of infection. Over the centuries since Jenner's time, doctors, health officials, and governments helped distribute the smallpox vaccine. The efforts largely freed rich countries of the disease. However, distributing the vaccine throughout the world required an unprecedented collaboration across countries. One man had a central role in the effort to eradicate the malady.

Donald A. Henderson, called "D. A." by all who knew him well, directed the program for the global eradication of smallpox. Although a physician, he did not vaccinate people, he did not see patients, and he did not develop new medical technology. What he did was organize and manage a huge army of people who worked in the field to identify those needing vaccines and to deliver the inoculations in a timely manner. He was the general who led the campaign.[8] Although managing an organization hardly seems heroic, public health success often depends on effective leadership to mobilize community action. Success must overcome opposition to public health measures, obtain adequate funding, and motivate workers to continue the difficult tasks they face in helping those in need. For smallpox eradication, public health success depended on what one colleague called Henderson's genius for management.[9]

The focus on Henderson and his accomplishments should not slight all the others involved. Henderson was the first to minimize his role and to give credit to others. He knew the success of the effort came from collaboration across countries and the actions of hundreds of thousands of people working in the field. Henderson can be seen as a representative of the larger public health effort. That said, one can agree with Richard Preston that "as much as anyone, D. A. Henderson was responsible for the eradication of smallpox."[10] The outcome "stands as one of the greatest accomplishments of the 20th century, if not one of the greatest human accomplishments of all time."[11] It is a model of public health success.

The World's Most Persistent and Feared Disease

Smallpox Shapes Human History

Although many infectious diseases have beset humans through history, smallpox stands out. Henderson described the horror of the disease:

> Smallpox, by far, [was] the most persistent and serious of all the pestilential diseases known to history . . . a disease that had maimed, blinded, and killed throughout the world since the dawn of written history. It was a disease more feared than any of the great pestilences—more than plague or yellow fever or cholera or malaria. It was a disease which virtually everyone eventually acquired.[12]

Smallpox frightened people in part because of its lethality. It spread widely through human contact, and about 30 percent of its victims died. It also frightened people because of its excruciating symptoms—a high fever and ugly, painful pustules that cover the body. The pustules are "hard pressurized blisters filled with a clear, faintly opalescent pus."[13] They produce a putrid smell and come with a fever high enough to make some victims delirious. Pustules inside the mouth and on the tongue make it difficult to eat and drink. Most survivors were left with deep scars over the face, and up to a third were left blind.[14] There was no treatment.

Smallpox is caused by the variola virus, which is transmitted from person to person. It enters the body when a person breathes in droplets from air containing the virus or allows the virus to enter the nose and mouth through contact with infected materials.[15] Although not a highly transmissible disease, it spreads readily where humans congregate closely, especially in densely populated settlements. Once inside the body, the virus enters and takes over cells to make copies of itself. It takes about ten to fourteen days after infection for a person to develop noticeable symptoms of a fever and aching pains. A rash and pustules appear a few days later. There are two types of the virus. The more deadly type, variola major, averages 30 percent mortality; variola minor has a mortality rate of less than 1 percent.[16]

Experts estimate that smallpox jumped from rodents to humans in northwestern Africa more than sixteen thousand years ago.[17] The first documented evidence, however, came from a mummified Egyptian pharaoh, whose face had indications of smallpox scars. The disease appears to have spread to India and China, where it has regularly victimized large parts of the population for more than two thousand years.[18] Smallpox so concerned people in parts of India that they created religious gods and temples devoted to protection from the disease. The Roman Empire inadvertently helped spread the infection by building roads that made it easier for travelers to carry the virus over long distances. It could then spread quickly through large Roman cities.[19]

Europe suffered from regular epidemics during the Middle Ages, terrifying populations with its suffering and death and filling churchyards with corpses.[20] The original term "variola," derived from Latin meaning "mark on the skin," changed to "smallpox" in England. The small "pocke," a term meaning "sac," distinguished the disease from the great pockes of syphilis.[21] The disease caused yet greater devastation when the Spanish brought it to the New World. Being previously unexposed to the disease and having no immunity, native populations died in enormous numbers, with death rates of 50–80 percent and entire tribes disappearing.[22] When the Pilgrims arrived at Plymouth Rock in 1620, the native population was already sparse owing to smallpox brought earlier by settlers in Nova Scotia.[23]

From Variolation to Vaccination

In 1721, Cotton Mather, a Puritan minister born in Boston, saw the devastation of smallpox firsthand. That year, a sailor on a British ship brought the disease to Boston. Despite efforts to quarantine the sailor, smallpox spread throughout the city. Boston had faced many outbreaks, but this one was the most serious: "Out of a population of 11,000, over 6,000 cases were reported with 850 dying from the disease."[24] Mather exhibited an odd mix of puritanical religious dogma and scientific perspective. He both supported the convictions of women in the Salem witchcraft trials of 1692–1693 and wrote scientific studies recognized for their quality throughout the United States and Europe. The spread of smallpox in 1721 stimulated his scientific side. A West African man he enslaved said that he was protected from smallpox by a simple procedure used in Africa. It involved taking material from a pustule of a smallpox victim and mixing a small amount into the blood of someone who had not had the disease. After reading about the procedure, Mather advocated its use in Boston, and a physician agreed to help. Of 287 people inoculated, only 2 percent died, compared with 14.9 percent among others.[25]

The information Mather found on the procedure came from an English aristocrat, Lady Mary Wortley Montagu. Her circumstances were much less dire than those suffering through the Boston outbreak. Lady Montagu had smallpox as a child and bore facial scars after recovering.[26] She was a lively, intelligent, and independent woman who impressed high society with her charm and writings.[27] Having gone to Turkey with her husband, the British ambassador, she heard of a smallpox-prevention procedure used by the court of the Ottoman Empire.[28] In 1718, Lady Montague tried the procedure by having the embassy surgeon insert smallpox material into her five-year-old son.[29] On her return to England in 1721, she did the same for her four-year-old daughter. All went well for the two children, who neither died from the inoculation nor became victims of the disease. She became a strong advocate of what was called "variolation," named after the variola virus.

Variolation turns out to have been used for thousands of years before becoming known in Europe and North America. Chinese physicians in the tenth century sought to create immunity by inserting material from smallpox lesions into the nasal passages.[30] Similar procedures in regions of Africa and India inserted the material into the skin. Entrance of the virus through the skin rather than through the nose and mouth appeared to reduce—but not eliminate—the risk of death.[31] It localized the infection and led to a mild form of the disease that nonetheless stimulated the production of antibodies. However, a small but meaningful percentage of children died as the result of being intentionally infected with the disease.

After successful tests using prisoners and orphans in London, variolation became accepted by many in the medical community and popular among the elite.[32] When the Princess of Wales variolated her daughters, the method became fashionable in English society. Foreshadowing conflict to come, however, some physicians viewed infecting children with smallpox as a form of murder.[33] The larger public did not like the idea either. One anti-variation opponent in Massachusetts, for example, was so angered that he threw a bomb through a window of Cotton Mather's house one night. The bomb came with a note: *"Cotton Mather, you dog, dam you! I'll inoculate you with this; with a pox to you."*[34]

The risks of variolation led decades later to development of the modern smallpox vaccine—perhaps the world's most successful vaccine. Edward Jenner, an English physician who was born in 1749, discovered, tested, and publicized an alternative to variolation. In so doing, he is commonly seen as the person responsible for one of the world's greatest lifesaving inventions. As a young child, he had undergone variolation treatment and remembered well the frightening fever and isolation he experienced.[35] While still a teen and apprenticing to a country doctor, Jenner learned of the common belief that dairymaids had beautiful complexions because they were protected from smallpox. He heard one dairymaid say, "I shall never have smallpox for I have had cowpox. I shall never have an ugly pockmarked face."[36] He wondered if cowpox, a disease common in cows that could be transferred to humans with little harm, might give people immunity from smallpox.

He bravely, perhaps unwisely, began an experiment. He took matter from cowpox lesions on the arms of a dairymaid and inoculated an eight-year-old boy, who developed a mild fever. Jenner then inoculated the boy with matter from a fresh smallpox lesion. The boy thankfully did not develop smallpox.[37] Jenner published a pamphlet in 1798 on his finding and gave the name vaccination to the procedure. In Latin, *vacca* refers to cow, *vaccinia* to cowpox, and, in Jenner's new terminology, "vaccination" referred to the produced immunity from cowpox. Jenner traveled throughout the world to demonstrate the technique and distribute the serum.[38] Historians found that others discovered the use of cowpox to confer immunity from smallpox before Jenner, but Jenner gets credit for researching and tirelessly promoting the use of vaccination.[39]

Vaccination spread rapidly through England, the United States, and most of Europe but also generated a good deal of fear and opposition. In 1853, legislation in England mandated that children be vaccinated by three months after birth. The law helped reduce smallpox but was not widely followed or enforced.[40] In addition to those not bothering with the vaccine as smallpox outbreaks declined, many actively objected. An influential anti-vaccination movement in the mid-1800s included notable intellectuals and diverse groups of followers.[41] In England, opponents went to the streets to protest compulsory vaccination, sometimes facing jail with the slogan "Better a felon's cell than a poisoned babe."[42] The opponents had diverse motives. Libertarians opposed government mandates, natural healing advocates saw the vaccine as unnatural, and sanitarian health authorities believed it detracted from the goal of clean cities. Those without ideological justification simply worried that it made healthy people sick. Pamphlets with titles such as *Vaccination, a Curse* and *Horrors of Vaccination* made outrageous claims, and misinformation about vaccines abounded.[43]

By the 1900s, persistent public health campaigns, advocacy from physicians and scientists, and favorable court rulings slowly overcame resistance. Britain had its last major smallpox outbreak in 1900–1905.[44] The illness largely disappeared thereafter from England, Europe, the United States, and Canada. Outbreaks occurred on occasion but usually arose from visitors bringing in the disease rather than from continuously present pockets of the virus.

People in less developed countries, however, had little access to vaccines and suffered from regular outbreaks of smallpox. By 1966, well into the twentieth century, smallpox remained endemic—or was found regularly—in thirty-three countries.[45] Around the world, up to 15 million cases occurred each year, with about one-third ending in death.[46] The death toll during the twentieth century is estimated to be about 300 million people, a number more than twice that from all military wars.[47]

The modern vaccine differs little from the one Jenner developed. It is a live rather than a deadened form of a disease, which until the 1950s required refrigeration. A crucial technological advance was the development of a freeze-dried vaccine that allowed long-term storage at ambient temperatures. The freeze-dried vaccine can be carried into tropical areas with little electrical power and refrigeration capacity. Technical advances meant little, however, without the organizational skill needed to deliver the vaccine to the hundreds of millions of people vulnerable to the disease.

The Failure and Promise of Eradication Campaigns

A Commitment to Surveillance

The life of D. A. Henderson lacks the drama of public health heroes who tramped through fever dens and cholera-infected neighborhoods or visited poor and sick residents in immigrant neighborhoods. His life was more akin to that of a commanding general and revered leader of an army of "150,000 pox-warriors."[48] He fought daily battles in meeting rooms, on the phone, and during travels to countries across the world to deal with problems and motivate public health workers. His opponents were politicians, bureaucrats, and organization leaders who did not share his vision for eradicating smallpox. Although less dramatic, his battles were as important as any to advancing global public health.

Born to an engineer father and nurse mother in 1928, Henderson enjoyed a pleasant, middle-class childhood in a suburb outside of Cleveland, Ohio. He attended nearby Oberlin College, where he met his wife-to-be, Nana Bragg. Having long admired an uncle who was a physician, Henderson decided early on a medical career.[49] He obtained a medical degree from the University of Rochester in upstate New York and then served his internship and residency at Mary Imogene Bassett Hospital in Cooperstown, New York.[50] He considered specializing in cardiology, but events forced a change.

Henderson expected that he would have to join the armed forces, where he likely would spend his time giving shots to new recruits. He learned that working for the Centers for Disease Control (CDC) offered an alternative to the military draft. The Epidemic Intelligence Service, a part of the CDC focused on stopping the spread of infectious diseases in the United States, had an open position for a physician. Henderson admitted that he had little interest in infectious diseases and no inkling of the importance smallpox would have in his life.[51] As part of his medical degree, he had written a paper on the 1833 cholera epidemic in Rochester. The paper had won a prize, which impressed the CDC hiring team and got him the job.[52] When the unit chief quit two months after Henderson started, a promotion followed.

Henderson found the work to be fascinating. He says, "I was soon captivated by the prospect of public health as a career."[53] Disease outbreaks were unique, interesting as a problem to solve, and involved high stakes. He viewed the Epidemic Intelligence Service as a medical fire department that must be ready to travel quickly in response to a disease outbreak. The chief of the epidemiology branch at the CDC, Dr. Alexander Langmuir, served as a mentor. Langmuir was "a legend in public health" who viewed careful surveillance and regular collection of data as a key to public health.[54] Henderson found Langmuir to be demanding and sometimes difficult, but also inspiring, creative, and an excellent teacher. In Langmuir's view, surveillance involved more than reading reports in an office. It involved shoe-leather epidemiology—leaving the office to personally investigate epidemics, collect data, talk to officials and patients, and partner with state and local officials. The strategy involved a mixture of scientific precision and practical application. Henderson's commitment to surveillance would continue well after he left the CDC to work for the global eradication of smallpox.

Henderson moved up the CDC ladder, becoming chief of the CDC's surveillance section. In this position, he could apply and fine-tune what he had learned about surveillance from Langmuir. Of special importance, he took charge of national preparations for the importation of smallpox into the United States and the outbreak of an epidemic.[55] He also served as an adviser on vaccination programs against smallpox and measles in West Africa.

A tall man with a powerful voice, Henderson was a fine storyteller who entertained friends and acquaintances with "a million stories about his life in public health."[56] He and his wife enjoyed entertaining, often with visitors from other countries.[57] Several traits suited him well for public health leadership. He had strong convictions, clear goals, and certainty of how to reach his goals.[58] That meant he was honest and forthright in presenting his opinions, which he communicated often and loudly.[59] "He did not hesitate to express his views—even if they were not shared by others."[60] The certainty he brought to difficult issues made him an effective leader, one whom others willingly followed. As one colleague said, "When he saw something was possible, he didn't give up. His absolute certainty about everything was an attribute as a leader."[61] These skills served him well throughout his career.

The Prospects for Smallpox Eradication

At the CDC, Henderson could take some satisfaction in how well public health organizations in the United States had controlled smallpox. Mass vaccination of children over past decades had largely eliminated the disease. In exceptional cases, when travelers imported the disease, the CDC and public health officials acted quickly to prevent its spread. A few visionaries proposed a program to eliminate smallpox in all countries across the world, including those in Africa, Asia, and South America where the disease was rampant. But most experts dismissed the idea. By the 1960s, no successful model of eradication existed, and respected biologists said the goal was unreachable.

The evidence seemed clear. Previous attempts to eradicate four diseases—hookworm, yellow fever, yaws, and malaria—had failed.[62] The most ambitious of the programs, malaria eradication, was launched in 1955 by the WHO. However, as Henderson writes, "By the mid-1960s, it was apparent to even the most optimistic that effective malaria control, let alone eradication, was beyond the reach of existing technology."[63] Despite an intensive commitment of human and financial resources, the program did not come close to its goal and was suspended in 1969.[64] The failures led to skepticism in the global health community about eradication programs. They were seen as too top heavy—directed from above and separated from the basic health services that national governments provided. Critics said that resources devoted to eradication detracted from primary health care.[65]

Despite resistance to the idea, Viktor Zhdanov, a virologist and deputy minister of health for the Soviet Union, proposed to the WHO World Health Assembly in 1958 that it undertake the global eradication of smallpox. The assembly approved the resolution but not because of its confidence in reaching the goal. Rather, it wanted to overcome Cold War hostilities by encouraging the full participation of the Soviet Union in the WHO and showing international solidarity.[66] Supporting the resolution offered a step toward cooperation.

The resolution, not surprisingly, failed to translate into committed action. The WHO devoted few resources to the program. The small-size budget and staff could make little if any headway against smallpox. The Soviet Union and other countries expressed frustration over the slow progress.[67] In 1965, after seven years, advocates of smallpox eradication, which by then included the United States as well as the Soviet Union, called for a stronger commitment with specific milestones.[68] The World Health Assembly directed the WHO director to develop a plan and a budget to eradicate the disease. The WHO would contribute $2.4 million, obtain donations from rich countries, and rely on funds from the budgets of nations participating in the eradication campaign.[69]

The proposal divided the assembly. Opponents said it was too ambitious, cost too much, and set an impossible goal. The director-general of the WHO, Marcelino Candau from Brazil, opposed the plan. He worried that the effort would fail and detract from his own commitment to malaria eradication.[70] After unusually long debate, the resolution passed by only two votes.[71]

Who would lead the effort? Director-General Candau wanted an American. Believing that the program would fail and resenting the advocacy of the United States for the program, he wanted an American to blame.[72] The American best suited to lead a program on smallpox eradication—and to take the blame for failure—was D. A. Henderson. He had a background in surveillance, led the anti-smallpox effort in the United States, and had consulted about smallpox control in other nations. As Henderson tells the story, "Assistant Surgeon General James Watt called me to Washington to inform me that I was being assigned to WHO in Geneva. I declined. . . . Watt told me that he had no choice but to order me to assume the directorship of the program for at least eighteen months."[73] The job required a move to Geneva, Switzerland, the location of WHO headquarters. Henderson and his family put their furniture in storage for a temporary overseas stay but would not see it again for eleven years.[74]

Problems to Overcome

Having been pressured to take the job, Henderson expected problems and difficulties in leading such an ambitious program. In fact, the challenges were greater than he realized, especially during the early years of his tenure.[75] He was thirty-eight years old, looked young, and lacked the maturity of other WHO leaders. He arrived in 1966 at the WHO headquarters in Geneva—a complex with spectacular views of the city and mountains—to a small, bare office and a tiny staff.[76] The eradication program headquarters, which supervised activities across dozens of countries, had only nine people at its very largest. Higher-ups at the WHO regularly rejected his requests for more staff. The meager resources reflected the negative view of the program held by the director-general.

At the start, the vast extent of the problem dwarfed the available resources. Henderson estimated that each year in the thirty-one endemic countries, there were 10 million to 15 million cases of smallpox.[77] About 2 million deaths occurred. More than 1 billion persons living in Brazil, most sub-Saharan African countries, India, Pakistan, Afghanistan, Nepal, and Indonesia risked catching the disease.[78] The program called for mass vaccination of 80 percent of the population, a level thought to lead to herd immunity.

The challenge appeared overwhelming. Delivering the vaccine to so many people in so many places depended on creativity and flexibility in dealing with the diverse politics, geography, religions, demographics, transportation, and program support across the countries.[79] Even measuring the extent of the problem and progress toward the goal was daunting. Having a background in health surveillance, Henderson wanted complete and accurate weekly reports from all countries with smallpox.[80] At the start, however, countries reported only 5 percent of actual cases.[81]

The problem was that most countries reported only the cases that came to the attention of authorities when victims visited health centers. That was not enough. Smallpox hid in out-of-the way places, small villages, urban slums, and homes of families wanting to avoid being quarantined. Surveillance required public health workers to search out victims, much like a detective, and accurately report their findings. Authorities needed to quickly collate and report the numbers. Only then could outbreaks be controlled and the extent of progress be tracked. Regrettably, local health officials often objected to the surveillance work. They wanted to report on vaccines delivered—something much easier to track. But Henderson knew that counting the numbers of vaccinated persons rather than the number of persons with smallpox missed the real target of the program.

The immense undertaking Henderson faced called for generous funding. Initially, the WHO contributed only $2.4 million. About 70 percent of the costs had to come from donations and health budgets of the countries with smallpox.[82] The program had to do its own fund-raising by convincing national politicians and health officials to contribute. Henderson noted that funding for prevention programs was more difficult to obtain than funding for clinical medicine.[83] The images of sick people and the efforts to save their lives had drama that preventing people from getting sick could rarely match.

Dealing with the bureaucracy of the WHO and national health ministries made funding problems worse. No organization other than the WHO could organize such a global public health effort—it had the necessary prestige and worldwide reach. At the same time, the eighty units and offices of the organization had become disjointed, rigid, and slow to make decisions.[84] The eradication program, in contrast, required speed and flexibility. Requests and questions had to go to the director-general who, given his dislike of the program, rarely responded. The WHO regional offices similarly ignored or openly opposed Henderson's initiatives.

A few examples illustrate the problem.[85] Mail from Henderson's central office to workers in the field had, according to protocol, to go through a regional office and a multistep approval process. It often took months to get a letter approved. Henderson worked around the bureaucracy by sending letters directly and quickly to field staff along with an official version that slowly moved through proper channels. Similarly, smallpox reporting initially had to proceed through official channels, often muddled by three reporting systems in a country. It took Henderson three years to persuade the WHO and member countries to allow people in the eradication program to report their numbers directly to his office. When the American government donated vehicles for program workers to use in traveling to remote areas, the WHO resisted using program funds for gasoline to fill their tanks. Equally frustrating was the insistence of Americans that the vehicles given to the program be American-made. Since few countries had the parts to repair American vehicles, program workers had to learn to repair breakdowns on their own.

The need for flexibility would seem obvious given the diversity of the countries with smallpox. Some had populations scattered across large areas and located in small and hard-to-reach villages. For example, smallpox in Indonesia endangered a population of 120 million that was dispersed across three thousand islands and 3,700 miles.[86] Nomadic populations moved from one place to another, crossing national borders and bringing smallpox with them. Some populations lived in dense urban settlements where smallpox victims hid away in places that outsiders could find only with difficulty. That each country had a different health care system added to the complexity of the problems.

Even with a carefully tailored plan for a country, unexpected events could quickly thwart progress. Over the years, the program worked in countries that suffered through droughts, floods, famine, other disease epidemics, washed-out roads, and communication breakdowns. Most problematic were coups, unstable governments, and civil wars that produced hordes of refugees and made soldiers suspicious of program workers. Civil wars in Nigeria, Pakistan, and Ethiopia obstructed public health activities and worsened the spread of smallpox. In some locations, eradication teams faced threats of arrest or kidnapping. Henderson wondered how he could plan and manage a program under such circumstances.[87]

The Importance of Management

Technological Innovation

Without his deep well of optimism and tenacity, Henderson might have given up right from the start. Never had such a large and difficult public health undertaking succeeded. He knew, however, that smallpox had several properties that made it a good candidate for eradication. Perhaps most important, the disease had lost the ability to survive outside of humans. Diseases that live in animals can jump across species and reinfect humans after apparent elimination. Similarly, asymptomatic diseases can hide and unknowingly be transmitted among humans. Smallpox victims, however, always had symptoms. Visible pustules made the presence of an infection relatively easy to identify. Another advantage was that the disease did not spread to others during the incubation period.[88] It spread at more advanced stages when the symptoms clearly showed, and people knew to stay away. And those exposed, if vaccinated soon enough, would not develop the disease.

Technological advances also contributed to the potential for eradication. The smallpox vaccine worked against all strains of smallpox, provided long-term immunity, and had few side effects. The freeze-dried form of the vaccine could be carried long distances and in hot weather without refrigeration. In 1965, a newly invented needle facilitated delivery of the vaccine. The bifurcated needle had two prongs, looked like a small olive fork, and allowed the vaccine to be inserted with light punctures of the skin. Vaccinators had no need for long needles and shots. They simply dipped the bifurcated needle in the vaccine and lightly punctured the upper arm multiple times in a small, circular area. A needle cost less than a penny and could be boiled and reused.[89] It used the vaccine solution sparingly—only one-quarter of traditional methods—and each vaccine cost only ten cents.[90] Vaccinators were trained in fifteen minutes with a 95 percent success rate and averaged five hundred vaccinations per day.[91]

Along with an efficient form of delivery, the vaccine itself must be of sufficient quality to produce immunity in recipients. Henderson found at first that only 10 percent of the vaccine batches met standards.[92] He implemented a testing protocol for vaccine quality and worked with labs to standardize production methods. The United States and the Soviet Union helped with generous donations of vaccine. Some labs refused to cooperate, but persistence paid off, with all vaccines meeting WHO standards by 1969.[93]

Key Principles

Technology would mean little without visionary leadership and effective management. Despite the complexity of the effort to work across dozens of nations, Henderson kept several key principles in mind as he guided the program.

The first was to emphasize clear and measurable objectives. Henderson set the goal of Target Zero—no smallpox cases. The

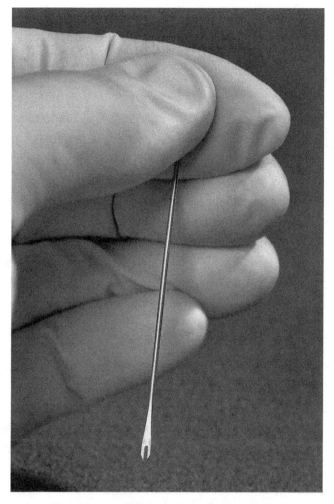

Bifurcated needle, which made inoculation with the smallpox vaccine
simple, efficient, and economical. *Source*: Wikimedia Commons, from the Centers
for Disease Control and Prevention.

slogan appeared on buildings, T-shirts, bumper stickers, and the
cover of WHO magazines. Staff members made toasts "To zero,"
and Henderson used the e-mail address DAHzero@aol.com.[94]
Henderson also displayed confidence in the ability reach the goal,
even with the inevitable obstacles, setbacks, and organizational

conflicts.[95] As a result, even local workers understood the importance of their work and their part in a huge global effort.[96]

The Target Zero goal helped counter desires to focus on the numbers vaccinated. The number of vaccinations, by itself, served only as a means to an end. The target of no smallpox cases directed workers to give vaccinations where they helped the most. The goal could then be specified in more concrete terms, such as "75% of outbreaks should be discovered within two weeks of the onset of the first case, that containment should begin within forty-eight hours, and that no new cases should occur more than seventeen days after containment had begun."[97]

The Target Zero goal relied on surveillance. Much as he did when working for the CDC, Henderson believed that success depended on watchfulness and reporting. Timely detection allowed for a timely response; slow reporting allowed the disease to spread before workers could respond with vaccinations. Officials supervising vaccination efforts sometimes penalized workers who reported smallpox cases. They wanted to show success in finding no cases.[98] Henderson defined success in terms of finding and responding to new cases. A system of reporting was put in place that rewarded citizens who reported cases. Where needed, "health personnel periodically swept through states searching every village and, eventually, every house during a 10-day period."[99]

A second guiding principle was delegation of authority to workers in the field. Henderson had little choice in the matter, as he had a tiny staff in Geneva, and many at the WHO headquarters and regional offices disapproved of the program. But he masterfully distributed responsibilities.[100] A flat management structure, with little in the way of hierarchy, allowed the Geneva staff to work around the layers of a formal bureaucracy and reach all the way to village health workers.[101] Far from being a micromanager, Henderson set goals but assigned responsibility to those in the field to find the best ways to reach them.[102] Management involved collegial discussion and persuasion and gave much latitude to the program's network of professional staff.

The WHO served more as a decentralized coordinating unit than a center of power.[103] Management in this case involved incessant communication with more than 700 lieutenants, 150 on loan from the CDC, who served in seventy-three countries.[104] Communication at the time lacked e-mail, cell phones, or the Internet and relied on the slow delivery of letters and uneven access to landline phones. Often isolated from headquarters, workers had to be independent and self-motivated. Henderson often spent time in the field, where he dealt directly with problems, devised solutions, and helped workers with their duties.[105] But workers learned how to get things done on their own.

The program staff proved amazingly innovative when given this freedom. In traveling into villages to search out cases, workers found that, with clear explanations of the importance of the tasks, village leaders enthusiastically helped with reporting and vaccinating.[106] In less populated areas, where residents were widely dispersed, workers had to find ways to identify outbreaks other than traveling from village to village. In Nigeria, a missionary-based radio network was used to get reports on cases.[107] In Ethiopia, people came regularly to markets from miles away, which offered an efficient way to find and respond to smallpox victims. Workers found, surprisingly, that schoolchildren knew much about smallpox outbreaks. One Indonesian worker turned in complete lists of smallpox cases with a few hours of effort. He said that he saved time by going to schools and talking to children ages eight to twelve years, who knew "almost everything that's going on in their own village and they are happy to share that information."[108] Elsewhere in Indonesia, workers found that showing a photo of baby with smallpox helped identify cases. Bus drivers, messengers, and military personnel who traveled across cities and regions helped report on cases.[109]

A third guiding principle emphasized collaboration and persuasion. The program depended on the cooperation of national and local leaders, and Henderson used a mix of science, politics, and personal relationships to build support for the program.[110] He skillfully negotiated global agreements and alliances and recruited a steady influx of skilled CDC workers to help with the program.[111] The cooperation of such a diverse and effective coalition of nations for a public health goal was indeed special.

The international prestige and the worldwide network of officials associated with the WHO, despite pockets of resistance, certainly contributed to the program's success. But Henderson's personal touch proved important to building the international collaboration. For example, in the face of conflict between the United States and the Soviet Union over leadership of the eradication program, Henderson invited Viktor Zhdanov, the Russian representative to the World Health Assembly, for a dinner of grilled steaks at the Henderson home in Geneva.[112] The relationship led to agreements on the need to improve vaccine quality and recruit better qualified staff from the Soviet Union. The amicable collaboration occurred despite Cold War hostilities between the two superpowers.[113]

A New Strategy

Surveillance-Containment

In 1966, Bill Foege, a physician and medical missionary in Nigeria, made a discovery that revolutionized the eradication campaign. Foege, tall and irrepressible, was on loan from the CDC.[114] A missionary colleague located in a remote Nigerian village used a shortwave radio to inform Foege of an outbreak.[115] Foege and a colleague rode ninety miles on small motorbikes to vaccinate residents of the village. On arriving, they confirmed five cases of smallpox. The protocol was to vaccinate everyone in the village, but because of a delay in the delivery of supplies, they lacked sufficient vaccine. They decided instead to vaccinate the immediate family members of the victims and those who had contact with the families. Forgoing mass vaccination of the village, they sought to protect those most susceptible.

Returning home from the village, Foege worried about new outbreaks among those he could not vaccinate. He was not hopeful. If smallpox returned to the village, then the targeted vaccination efforts had been wasted. Because the village lacked telephones, Foege turned on his shortwave radio each night to check on reports of smallpox cases. To his "joy and amazement," the disease had not spread beyond the initial isolated cases.[116]

Foege realized he had made a groundbreaking discovery. Mass vaccination of villages, towns, cities, and countries was inefficient, even unnecessary. In one city, he and others had managed to vaccinate 94 percent of the residents, but smallpox still emerged among a small group that had been missed.[117] The alternative, vaccinating those who had been exposed to the virus through contact with a victim exhibiting symptoms, worked much better. The strategy is often called "ring vaccination." It required a rapid response that created a ring of vaccinated persons around smallpox patients. Once limited to inside the ring and unable to jump to a new unvaccinated host, the virus would die out from the area. Foege used an apt metaphor to explain the logic of this method: "If a house is on fire, no one wastes time putting water on nearby houses just in case the fire spreads. They rush to pour water where it will do the most good—on the burning house. The same strategy turned out to be effective in eradicating smallpox."[118]

Foege and his team received permission to further test the new strategy. Ring vaccination worked because, they discovered, smallpox spread relatively slowly.[119] Victims infected others through face-to-face contact in enclosed spaces such as homes, schools, and hospitals only during the last stages of the illness. In most cases, those exposed to the disease could be located and vaccinated while it was still incubating in their bodies. The vaccination then prevented further spread. The strategy depended on accurate reporting and a quick, intense response. A ring had to be created quickly before smallpox could infect others.

Henderson, always open to new ideas and contrarian views, recognized the value of the new approach.[120] He called it "eradication-escalation,"[121] but another name, "surveillance-containment," emphasized the key components of reporting and vaccination response. Beginning in 1967, the eradication program shifted its strategy away from mass vaccination.[122] Targeted actions proved more efficient and more effective. Foege believed that with surveillance and containment as the primary strategy, mass vaccination became a wasted effort and could be dropped totally.[123]

With the new strategy, intense surveillance took on even more importance than it had previously possessed.[124] To stop smallpox transmission, workers had to know where outbreaks occurred. Mobile surveillance teams regularly visited designated areas to search for smallpox cases. Whenever possible, the surveillance teams operated separately from the vaccination teams, which tended to focus on counts of vaccinations rather than on smallpox cases. In Brazil, for example, setting up more than three thousand reporting posts greatly improved on past practices of relying on reports from officials at state capitals and a few major cities.[125]

Demonstrating the effectiveness of surveillance-containment in Nigeria did not always go easily.[126] National and local health authorities initially offered little support. They distrusted a targeted approach that left large parts of the population unvaccinated. Worse, the Biafran civil war in the country meant that armed soldiers often stopped teams at roadblocks as they traveled to villages to find and respond to new outbreaks. In one city, police arrested Foege as he scouted for locations where large crowds could be vaccinated; he spent six hours in jail. In another part of the country, he was put under house arrest for four days and then forced to leave the country.

Despite the problems, the surveillance-containment strategy succeeded in eastern Nigeria, where Foege was located. Smallpox surprisingly had disappeared within five months. Foege was shocked at the quick results, even though only 750,000 of 12 million were vaccinated.[127] Henderson observed equally successful tests in other nations.[128] In Sierra Leone, a country with the highest smallpox incidence rate in the world in 1967 and 1968, the disease disappeared in eight months, even though only 70 percent of the country had been vaccinated. In Central Java, an Indonesian province of 28 million, only 50,000 vaccinations succeeded in ending transmissions after eight months.

Extending the surveillance-containment strategy to other countries in western and central Africa meant dealing with the regular movement of people and groups across borders. The eradication campaign had to target a contiguous bloc of twenty countries with a combined population of 120 million.[129] Each had different governments, languages, economies, topographies, religions, tribal loyalties, and population densities. After giving priority to surveillance-containment and with the contribution of staff and funds from the CDC,[130] smallpox disappeared from the area by May 1970, about three and a half years later.[131] Progress had occurred substantially more quickly than anticipated.[132] As one US surgeon general commented, the enthusiastic and energetic workers were "simply too young to realize they couldn't do it."[133]

Struggles in East Asia

Success in western Africa provided the boost to morale needed to keep the eradication campaign moving forward. Indeed, a good dose of confidence facilitated the campaign in India, Bangladesh, and surrounding countries. These populous nations with more than 700 million people were more densely packed than those in most of western Africa. The population density made the disease hard to locate and easy to spread. Beginning in 1962, Indian officials had launched an ambitious program that over the next four years vaccinated around 440 million people.[134] Still, disease outbreaks occurred often. In 1967, 65 percent of all reported smallpox cases in the world occurred in India.[135]

Dealing with such large and densely packed populations multiplied the potential for explosive transmission of the virus. Advocates of the surveillance-containment strategy wondered if it would work in such difficult circumstances. In one area of India in 1974, for example, 11,600 new cases were reported in a single week.[136] Finding all the new cases, many hidden away in slum areas and villages, required tiring and slow house-to-house searches.[137] Sometimes it required use of all the senses. Foege tells of his experiences:

> On at least two occasions, smell alone alerted me to the presence of smallpox. As I walked down a hospital hallway in India, the dead-animal odor stopped me in my tracks; following the smell, I located a smallpox patient. Another time, as I walked down an alley in an urban slum in Pakistan, the same smell hit me. There are competing smells in such places, but again one smell stood out. Knocking on doors, I found two siblings with smallpox.[138]

Although somewhat apprehensive, Henderson moved forward with the surveillance-containment strategy. With support from the prime minister of India, Indira Gandhi, an army of vaccinators was mobilized.[139] First, however, search teams needed to measure the extent of the problem and identify locations where the vaccinators should concentrate their efforts. The zealous efforts of the search teams found unexpectedly and discouragingly high numbers of cases, even in places where smallpox was thought to be rare.[140] As surveillance improved, reports showed higher rather than lower numbers of smallpox cases. Although the actual number of smallpox cases may have been declining, it appeared to outsiders that things were getting worse.

India had a large and complex health bureaucracy that some- times interfered as much as helped. In one Indian state, the min- ister of health responded to pressure from legislators and politi- cians by halting the surveillance-containment strategy after only seven months.[141] The minister wanted to return to the mass vac- cination strategy that had failed over the past century to make much of a dent in smallpox prevalence. Only at the last minute did he allow his workers to continue with the strategy for another month. Fortunately, one more month was all that was needed to show progress.

Citizens rarely refused to be vaccinated, but many were hard to find. Vaccinators had to take a census of exposed households to ensure containment.[142] Even then, keeping smallpox patients iso- lated from the unvaccinated presented problems. Despite a goal to maintain a six-foot perimeter between the patient and susceptible people, sympathetic visitors from all around followed local norms to console the victim. Guards had to be hired and placed at each patient's home with instructions to vaccinate every visitor.[143]

Progress advanced slowly but steadily. The last reported case in India occurred in May 1975. As Foege summarized, "In twenty months, the surveillance/containment approach had proved itself ideally suited for eradicating a virus that had eluded the best ef- forts of mass vaccination programs for 175 years. It was the right tool for the task."[144] Similar progress occurred in the nearby coun- tries of Nepal and Bangladesh, again after persistence in dealing with major disasters. Bangladesh, part of Pakistan at the start of the eradication campaign, fought a civil war and gained independence in 1971. However, the civil war and disastrous floods brought streams of refugees across the border into India. After independence, refugees returned to their new country, bringing smallpox with them.[145] In 1975, intensified reporting and vaccination efforts plus isolation of patients with armed guards involved 112,000 workers in the field every day.[146]

The last case of variola major in the world occurred in Bangladesh in October 1975 with the infection of a three-year-old girl named Rahima Banu. To contain a potential outbreak, a team came by boat, motorcycle, and foot to the island where the family of the victim lived. After quarantining the family and vaccinating eighteen thousand people living within one mile, the offer of a reward failed to uncover any new cases.[147] By January 1976, smallpox had been eradicated from Asia.

Last Cases in Ethiopia and Somalia

Despite eliminating variola major, the deadliest form of the disease, variola minor, still a serious form of smallpox, remained in one eastern African country—Ethiopia. Outbreaks occurred in the mountain highlands, where workers traveled by mules on the winding trails or by helicopters to fly to local villages.[148] A drought and famine plus a rebellion led the refugees to migrate and spread the disease. Rebels overthrew the existing government in 1974, and civil disorder in the country forced the United States to remove volunteers.[149] The new government fortunately allowed the eradication program to move forward. An assist came from a donation of $1 million by the US surgeon general to purchase three helicopters to reach difficult areas.[150] The helicopters sometimes attracted unwanted attention in the villages, including rifle shots, forced landings, and one hostage situation.[151] Even so, the eradication team there saw steady progress.

But things took a turn for the worse with the discovery of smallpox cases in neighboring Somalia. The government there had

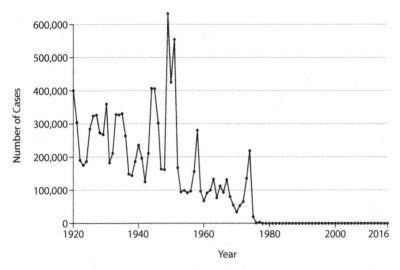

Global number of reported smallpox cases, 1920–2016. In December 1979, the disease was officially declared eradicated worldwide. *Source*: Wikimedia Commons, adapted from Our World in Data. Creative Commons CC BY 4.0.

been suppressing reports of outbreaks.[152] Henderson noted his bitter disappointment at the new cases just as they were nearing success everywhere else.[153] The problem in Somalia came from a population of herders who traveled long distances, often moving across borders, in search of land for grazing. The migrants were hard to track, but once again, the surveillance-containment strategy worked. The last case occurred on October 26, 1977, with the hunt for and isolation of Ali Maow Maalin. Variola minor, like variola major, had disappeared from the natural world. The eradication campaign led by Henderson had met its goal, only nine months past the original ten-year target.[154]

Ongoing Global Vaccination

In December 1979, after more than two years of waiting and checking for other cases, an independent global commission meeting in Nairobi, Kenya, declared that smallpox had been erad-icated.[155] The commission further recommended that all small-pox vaccinations cease—the disease was no longer a threat. In a ceremony in Nairobi, the WHO director-general declared, "Oc-tober 26 shall henceforth be designated as 'Smallpox Zero' day—a day of remembrance and reaffirmation of the achievement possi-ble when peoples everywhere band together, without regard to politics or national glory, in pursuit of a common goal."[156] A statue dedicated to the eradication of smallpox stands in front of the WHO headquarters in Geneva.[157]

Reflecting on his eleven years leading the smallpox eradication program, Henderson admitted that victory over the disease was reached by the thinnest of margins. "Smallpox eradication proved to be infinitely more difficult than I or anyone else had imagined it would be."[158] The program had to overcome a daunting set of problems but also benefited from some fortunate events:

> floods, wars and famines, hundreds of thousands of refugees, national bureaucracies and constraints that rivalled the US in number and complexity, a difficult USAID programme (an unwilling but a significant contributor), and a sclerotic WHO administration that often thwarted or actively impeded what appeared to be logical initiatives . . . changes in governments, fortuitous laboratory discover-ies, unexpected successes in launching vaccine production operations in developing country laboratories, and the emergence of needed leadership and courage by national and international staff at numerous critical points.[159]

Henderson ended his career at the WHO with the successful completion of the eradication goal. He felt both joyful and sad—joyful because of the extraordinary accomplishment of the pro-gram and sad because of the end of his collaboration with "as ex-traordinary and as dedicated a group of people as any with whom

I have ever worked."[160] While admittedly a grind, his time as leader of the project turned out to be enormously satisfying. William Foege felt much the same. Over a career that included heading the CDC and working with the Gates Foundation, he recalled his time in Africa and India as the highlight of his life: "I had been immersed in helping to solve a problem of great importance, working alongside people of superb abilities and motivations. The hardships were overshadowed by the blessings."[161]

In 1977, Henderson moved to a new job as dean of what is now the Johns Hopkins Bloomberg School of Public Health.[162] He again thrived as a leader and manager. Of special note, he revised the public health curriculum in order to send more students into the field and emphasize practical experience along with academics. After thirteen years, he resigned as dean to serve in the President's Office of Science and Technology in Washington, DC, and then in the Office of the Secretary of Health and Human Services.[163] Having become an expert on bioterrorism, he advised several presidents on national responsiveness. In 1998, he founded and directed the Johns Hopkins Center for Civilian Biodefense Strategies, and after September 11, 2001, he directed the Office of Public Health Emergency Preparedness in the Department of Health and Human Services.[164]

For the rest of his life, Henderson worried about a new risk created by the eradication program. Although naturally occurring smallpox had disappeared, several research labs kept samples for scientific purposes. The storage issue quickly ran into problems. In 1978, the virus escaped from a lab at the Birmingham Medical School in England, where it killed a forty-year-old photographer, Janet Parker.[165] Immediate vaccination of her contacts, five hundred in total, prevented the spread of the disease. Henderson favored destroying all stocks of the virus, but others wanted to keep some for genomic analysis. The WHO decided to allow two labs, one at the Moscow Research Institute of Viral Preparations and one at the CDC in Atlanta, to keep the virus under rigorous safety conditions.[166]

Henderson knew that ending vaccinations made new generations vulnerable to use of the disease as a bioterrorist weapon. Evidence suggested that the Soviet Union had sought to create large amounts of smallpox as a biological weapon.[167] In lieu of destroying all smallpox samples, Henderson successfully advocated for the creation of a national stockpile of smallpox vaccine.[168]

Henderson died in 2016 at age eighty-seven from complications of a hip fracture. By that time, he had received the Presidential Medal of Freedom, National Medal of Science, National Academy of Sciences Public Welfare Medal, and many others.[169] As a physician, Henderson differed from the norm. "His house calls were to villages, smallpox wards, prime ministers, and presidents."[170] His work "inspired public health students and practitioners worldwide and embodies the spirit of global health for millions of people."[171]

After his experience leading the only successful campaign to eradicate a worldwide disease, Henderson expressed pessimism about the eradication of other diseases. The difficulty of the smallpox eradication program and the narrow escape from failure time and time again warranted some skepticism about future efforts. Partly in jest, but also reflecting his views about public health, Henderson often said that bad management should be eradicated next.[172]

The success of the smallpox program nonetheless motivated leaders to expand global vaccination initiatives. In 1974, the WHO sponsored national vaccination programs for DPT (diphtheria, pertussis, and tetanus), polio, and measles. The Expanded Program on Immunization succeeded by 1990 in its goal to vaccinate 80 percent of the world's children against these diseases.[173] Other diseases added to the program included rubella and yellow fever. Although not eradicated, these diseases currently kill fewer people worldwide than ever before.[174]

Today, the Global Polio Eradication Initiative, a public-private partnership that includes the WHO, the CDC, and the Gates Foundation, follows the surveillance and vaccination strategy used against smallpox. The initiative's webpage lists two countries where the disease remains endemic (Afghanistan and Pakistan), seven countries at risk because of low levels of immunity and surveillance, and twenty-eight countries experiencing outbreaks owing to importation of the disease from elsewhere.[175] The figures reflect remarkable progress. Cases worldwide have fallen from 350,000 in 1988 to 1,226 in 2020.[176] The CDC estimates that 18 million people who are currently healthy would have been paralyzed by polio without the program.[177]

Henderson viewed these vaccination efforts as the chief public health legacy of the smallpox eradication program.[178] But another legacy follows: organizational leadership and effective management are crucial components of successful public health programs. The eradication campaign, like many other public health projects, depended as much on persuasion as on science, as much on an organization such as the WHO as on the vaccine itself.[179] The momentous public health success against smallpox came from cooperation involving Henderson in Geneva; Foege and other leaders in Nigeria, India, and elsewhere; and an army of field workers in countries across the world.

Epilogue

In 2020, Johan Mackenbach, a Dutch physician and professor of public health, published a 442-page book, *A History of Population Health*, that describes the long-term changes in health and mortality in Europe since the 1700s.[1] It's a monumental effort to present and make sense of the patterns of change across diverse countries, time periods, and causes of death. The numerous graphs, tables, and figures are impressively detailed. The work reflects Mackenbach's view that public health is the most exciting field of science "because of the intellectual and practical challenges that we're facing."[2]

The centuries-long perspective offered by the book reveals just how astounding the progress against disease and death has been. Life expectancy at birth in Europe averaged only around forty years in the mid-1800s. Since then, it has risen rapidly and now ranges from sixty-five to eighty years for men and from seventy-five to eighty-five years for women.[3] In the United States in 2020, average life expectancy was seventy-five years for men and eighty-one years for women.[4] Much of the improvement came from eliminating deaths during childhood—a miracle for parents who suffered through the all-to-common loss of a child. Steven Johnson notes that the improvements in life expectancy have given the average adult about twenty thousand additional days of living—a whole extra life compared to hundreds of years ago.[5] As Mackenbach states, "It is difficult to think of a more important change in the whole of human history—unimaginable even for the most utopian among our predecessors."[6]

In one part of the book, Mackenbach presents what he admits is a "heroic exercise" to attribute the reductions in mortality to public health efforts and medical care.[7] While the estimates are far from certain, the exercise helps organize a good deal of historical data. During the early stages of the transition in Europe from high mortality in preindustrial societies to low mortality in postindustrial societies, Mackenbach finds that public health had a primary role. Public health measures were the dominant source of early reductions in plague, smallpox, and typhus and later had a major role in reductions in cholera, respiratory tuberculosis, syphilis, and childhood infections. More recently, public health had a major role in reducing deaths from lung cancer, liver cirrhosis, and traffic accidents. Mackenbach summarizes his findings by saying, "These results show that, over time, medical care has become much more important for mortality decline, but that over the three centuries covered by this book public health has been the most important of the two."[8] He states further that "it is impossible to escape the conclusion that some form of goal-directed 'human agency' played a crucial role."[9]

The seven people covered in this book illustrate the importance of goal-directed human agency for improvements in health. Their actions alone did not produce widespread change. Improvements in health can be seen as akin to social movements for universal suffrage or the abolition of slavery.[10] The movements involved the large-scale reshaping of how people lived and the political and social institutions that guided social life. Nonetheless, these seven key actors served as catalysts for larger public health movements.

Several themes emerge from the lives and accomplishments of the public health innovators.

1. All seven contributed to the progress against death and disease by helping to mobilize the community action that characterizes the field of public health. Harvey Wiley, Lillian Wald, and D. A. Henderson organized armies of donors, supporters, volunteers, and workers to promote public health. Edwin Chadwick, John Snow, W. E. B. Du Bois, and Richard Doll provided the data to rally support for sanitation, clean water, racial equality, and antismoking regulations. Although public support was hard-won it eventually enabled advances in public health to occur. The public health advocates helped make health a matter of "social as well as individual responsibility."[11]

2. Many of the historical advances in public health depended in good part on the regular and systematic collection and analysis of data. Although John Snow was much more skilled in the analysis of data than Edwin Chadwick, both used statistics to make their case for clean streets and clean water. Harvey Wiley relied on data from chemical analyses and a controversial experiment. W. E. B. Du Bois carried out an early study of social conditions and health. Richard Doll and colleagues presented new ways of understanding the causes of smoking-related disease through data collection and analysis. D. A. Henderson made surveillance of disease and the quick reporting of data the key to the success in eradicating smallpox. The gathering and analysis of data that defines epidemiology today has been critical to public health success dating back at least two hundred years.

3. Success in improving the health of the public required sustained effort. Entrenched interests—businesses wanting to increase profits, politicians seeking to maintain power, and parts

of the public relying on traditional but misguided beliefs about health—made progress difficult. Against daunting odds, all seven kept pushing to reach their goals. Edwin Chadwick's career consisted in good part of bureaucratic infighting. John Snow, in his calm, steady, and scientific way, disputed the dominant medical beliefs about the miasmatic spread of disease. It took Harvey Wiley nearly twenty-five years as a government chemist to reach his goal of federal food safety legislation. Lillian Wald and Richard Doll devoted all their adult lives to their public health goals, and W. E. B. Du Bois committed the whole of his mature life to the goal of racial equality in health and social life. D. A. Henderson, during the eleven years he headed the global eradication of smallpox program, had to overcome nearly overwhelming political and organizational obstacles.

4. All seven sought to improve the health of the public by targeting groups in special need and addressing problems of social inequality. The filth and impure water in London at the time of Edwin Chadwick and John Snow affected the lives of what were known as the laboring classes—those who could not afford a clean neighborhood and safe water. Lillian Wald sought to help the destitute immigrants living in New York City, and W. E. B. Du Bois sought to help oppressed African Americans in Philadelphia. D. A. Henderson protected billions of poor people in South America, Africa, and Asia. Harvey Wiley and Richard Doll helped bring about changes that promoted food safety and nonsmoking that, while benefiting all social strata, addressed problems of special severity among less advantaged groups. All the innovators, to varying degrees, recognized poverty as a social cause of disease and loss of life, and though they could do little to address the root causes, believed that policies could help those in need. Addressing inequalities in health remains a central part of the public health agenda today.[12]

5. Public health success depended on legislation and political action. Sometimes change came from mobilizing public support (Harvey Wiley), sometimes from working directly with legislators and government officials (Edwin Chadwick, Lillian Wald, D. A. Henderson), and sometimes from relying on scientific evidence to change opinions of politicians and the public (John Snow, W. E. B. Du Bois, Richard Doll). Bringing about improvements in the health of the public depended in good part on political success.

The themes common throughout the history of public health apply to the new challenges faced by the field in the twenty-first century. The previous chapters describe the legacy of public health advocates in the efforts to safely dispose of human waste in poor areas of the world; to ensure safe drinking water; to protect the public from dangerous food; to serve the public outside of hospitals, clinics, and physician's offices; to advance the ongoing battle for racial equality; to eliminate the harmful use of tobacco; and to extend global vaccination programs. Applying lessons of the past to the present is seldom a simple process, but knowing about the public health innovators of the past can offer encouragement in dealing with current problems.

The same themes apply today as public health confronted the outbreak and spread of the coronavirus disease (COVID-19) caused by the SARS-CoV-2 virus. Community action in response to the virus took forms we have all come to know well: restricting indoor gatherings and outdoor crowds, limiting face-to-face business activity, isolating the sick, wearing masks, maintaining social distance, testing for the virus, and providing vaccinations.[13] A good deal of effort has gone into protecting the most vulnerable— the elderly and those with preexisting health problems. The use of data and surveillance has been crucial, as local, national, and worldwide figures on infections and deaths were updated daily.

Policies today, as in the past, depend on accurate, consistent, and reliable statistics.[14] Also as in the past, the heroes of the COVID-19 pandemic are contested, as are many of the policies. The kinds of battles fought by the seven people in this book to improve public health will continue, but because of the battles, so will the progress.

ACKNOWLEDGMENTS

I would like to thank my editor, Robin Coleman, and the anonymous reviewers who provided helpful comments on earlier drafts of the manuscript. My wife, Jane, kindly edited each chapter in the early stages of writing, and Beth Gianfagna and Kyle Kretzer improved the manuscript with editing in the final stages of manuscript preparation. And I owe many thanks to all those who, along with the seven people highlighted in this book, contributed to the amazing advances in public health over the last several centuries. We have all benefited from their accomplishments.

NOTES

Introduction

1. Pflaumer 2015, 2666.
2. UK National Archives 2021.
3. McKeown and Record 1962, 104, calculations from table 3.
4. McKeown and Record 1962, 110.
5. Colgrave 2002, 728.
6. Johnson 2021a, 33.
7. McKeown 1976a, 1976b; McKeown and Brown 1955; Szreter 1988, 5.
8. Winslow 1920, 30.
9. Berridge 2016, 2.
10. Teutsch and Fielding 2013, 287.
11. Porter 1998, 1-2.
12. Johnson 2021b.

Chapter 1. The Obnoxious Bureaucrat

1. Brundage 1988, 131.
2. Hamlin 1998, 183.
3. Brundage 1988, 130-131.
4. Hardy 1999, 255.
5. Poynter 1962, 382.
6. Finer 1952, 10.
7. Brundage 1988, 132.
8. Hamlin and Sheard 1998, 588.
9. Listios 2003, 189.
10. M. White 2009.
11. Marston 1925, 98.
12. Bryson 2010, 419.
13. Chadwick 1842, 47.

14. M. Henderson 2011.
15. M. White 2009.
16. Jackson 2014, 105-106.
17. Bryson 2010, 421.
18. Rosen [1958] 2015, 114.
19. Rosen [1958] 2015, 112.
20. Flinn 1965, 14.
21. Flinn 1965, 15.
22. Finer 1952, 10.
23. Finer 1952, 9.
24. Finer 1952, 10.
25. Finer 1952, 19.
26. Hempel 2007, 115.
27. Brundage 1988, 4; Finer 1952, 3-4; Hempel 2007, 115; Marston 1925, 92.
28. Conniff 2014.
29. Chadwick quoted in Phillips 2003, 97.
30. Finer 1952, 2.
31. Finer 1952, 2.
32. Finer 1952, 2.
33. Finer 1952, 5.
34. Brundage 1988, 157.
35. Finer 1952, 513.
36. Marston 1925, 20.
37. Marston 1925, 20-21.
38. Chadwick 1828, 1.
39. Phillips 2003, 97.
40. Finer 1952, 16.
41. Finer 1952, 31.
42. Marston 1925, 18.

43. Bentham 1776, 1.
44. Finer 1952, 35.
45. Brundage 1988, 8.
46. Finer 1952, 39.
47. Brundage 1988, 20.
48. Rosen [1958] 2015, 107.
49. Halliday 2001, 1469.
50. Halliday 2001, 1469.
51. Hamlin 1996, 236.
52. Marston 1925, 41.
53. Marston 1925, 155.
54. Rosen [1958] 2015, 108.
55. Brundage 1988, 20.
56. Marston 1925, 174.
57. Poor Law Commission 1834, 262.
58. Rosen [1958] 2015, 111.
59. Poor Law Commission 1834, 295, 297.
60. Jackson 2014, 71.
61. Hamlin and Sheard 1998, 588.
62. Corbett 1999, 381.
63. Brundage 1988, 10.
64. Brundage 1988, 54.
65. Dickens quoted in Brundage 1988, 97.
66. Brundage 1988, 79.
67. Poynter 1962, 381.
68. Poynter 1962, 386.
69. Poynter 1962, 387, 389.
70. Poynter 1962, 384.
71. Gordon 1897.
72. Gordon 1897.
73. Smith quoted in Brown 2008, 531.
74. Brundage 1988, 96.
75. Listios 2003, 189.
76. Powell quoted in Poynter 1962, 390.
77. Hamlin 1998, 120.
78. Brundage 1988, 130.
79. Chadwick quoted in Brundage 1988, 131.
80. Chadwick quoted in Brundage 1988, 131.
81. Chadwick quoted in Brundage 1988, 132.
82. Rosen [1958] 2015, 116.
83. Finer 1952, 157.
84. Finer 1952, 158.
85. Flinn 1965, 18.
86. Flinn 1965, 21.
87. Hamlin 1998, 21.
88. Hamlin 1998, 49.
89. Hamlin 1988, 88.
90. Jackson 2014, 69.
91. Marston 1925, 93.
92. Brundage 1988, 80.
93. Flinn 1965, 45.
94. Flinn 1965, 45.
95. Hamlin 1996, 234.
96. Hamlin 1996, 234.
97. Flinn 1965, 37.
98. Hamlin 1998, 12–13.
99. Flinn 1965, 47.
100. Questionnaire quoted in Flinn 1965, 48.
101. Flinn 1965, 51.
102. Finer 1952, 212.
103. Finer 1952, 212.
104. Queijo 2010, 42.
105. Finer 1952, 339.
106. Flinn 1965, 2.
107. Flinn 1965, 35.
108. Finer 1952, 210.
109. Lewis quoted in Finer 1952, 210.
110. Finer 1952, 210.
111. Flinn 1965, 26.
112. Chadwick 1842, 3.
113. Chadwick 1842, 369.
114. Chadwick 1842, 5.
115. Chadwick 1842, 6.
116. Chadwick 1842, 11.
117. Chadwick 1842, 40.

118. Chadwick 1842, 42.
119. Chadwick 1842, 26–27.
120. Chadwick 1842, 30.
121. Marshall quoted in Chadwick 1842, 80.
122. Marshall quoted in Chadwick 1842, 80.
123. Marshall quoted in Chadwick 1842, 80.
124. Quoted in Chadwick 1842, 91.
125. Chadwick 1842, 107.
126. Chadwick 1842, 98.
127. Chadwick 1842, 370.
128. Quoted in Chadwick 1842, 99.
129. Byles quoted in Chadwick 1842, 148.
130. Chadwick 1842, 44.
131. Chadwick 1842, 48.
132. Chadwick 1842, 48.
133. Flinn 1965, 61.
134. Finer 1952, 221.
135. Flinn 1965, 61.
136. Chadwick 1842, 53.
137. Chadwick 1842, 63.
138. Chadwick 1842, 77.
139. Chadwick 1842, 371.
140. Chadwick 1842, 371.
141. Chadwick 1842, 341.
142. Flinn 1965, 62.
143. Chadwick 1842, 372.
144. Chadwick 1842, 371.
145. Hamlin 1998, 153–154.
146. Hamlin 1998, 163.
147. Flinn 1965, 70.
148. Hamlin and Sheard 1998, 587.
149. Fee and Brown 2005, 866.
150. Fee and Brown 2005, 867.
151. Fee and Brown 2005, 867.
152. Marston 1925, 114.
153. Fee and Brown 2005, 867.
154. Finer 1952, 468.
155. Finer 1952, 224.

156. Brundage 1988, 135.
157. Jackson 2014, 97.
158. Hardy 1999, 256.
159. World Health Organization 2022.
160. B. Gates 2021.
161. Queijo 2010, 31.

Chapter 2. The Disease Detective
1. Cameron and Jones 1983, 393.
2. Vinten-Johansen et al. 2003, 10.
3. Hempel 2013b, 1269.
4. Quoted in Hempel 2013b, 1269.
5. Condrau and Worboys 2007, 149.
6. Cameron and Jones 1983, 393.
7. Ball 2009, 110.
8. S. Snow 2008, 23.
9. John Snow Society 2020.
10. Shapin 2006.
11. Hempel 2013b.
12. McNeil 2019.
13. LiveScience Staff 2009.
14. Pollitzer 1954, 421–423.
15. Hamlin 2009, 46.
16. Pollitzer 1954, 430.
17. S. Snow 2002, 908.
18. Ball 2009, 109.
19. Pollitzer 1954, 458–459.
20. Condrau and Worboys 2007, 149.
21. Shapin 2006.
22. S. Snow 2002, 908.
23. Ball 2009, 106.
24. Hamlin 2009, 2.
25. Shapin 2006.
26. Rosenberg 1966, 455.
27. World Health Organization 2019.
28. Johnson 2006, 16.
29. Johnson 2006, 17–19.

30. Johnson 2006, 21–22.
31. Frerichs, n.d., "Index Case at 40 Broad Street."
32. Frerichs, n.d., "Reverend Henry Whitehead."
33. Snow quoted in Frerichs, n.d., "Broad Street Pump Outbreak."
34. S. Snow 2000a, 27–29.
35. Ellis 1994, xii.
36. Ellis 1994, x.
37. S. Snow 2000a, 30.
38. Ellis 1994, x.
39. S. Snow 2000b, 71.
40. Richardson [1866] 1952, 267.
41. S. Snow 2000b, 72.
42. S. Snow 2000b, 72.
43. Ellis 1994, xiii.
44. Richardson [1866] 1952, 268.
45. Richardson [1866] 1952, 267.
46. Wootton 2006, 198.
47. Vinten-Johansen et al. 2003, 40.
48. S. Snow 2000b, 73.
49. Richardson [1866] 1952, 270, 285.
50. Richardson [1866] 1952, 270.
51. Richardson [1866] 1952, 286.
52. Richardson [1866] 1952, 285–288.
53. Ellis 1994, xiii.
54. Vinten-Johansen et al. 2003, 24.
55. Ellis 1994, xv.
56. S. Snow 2000b, 73.
57. S. Snow 2000b, 75.
58. Vinten-Johansen et al. 2003, 237.
59. John Snow Archive and Research Companion, n.d., "John Snow's Published Works."
60. S. Snow 2000b, 76.
61. John Snow Archive and Research Companion, n.d., "On Asphyxia."
62. Vinten-Johansen et al. 2003, 5.
63. S. Snow 2000b, 77.
64. Ball 2009, 106.
65. Paneth 2004, 515.
66. Richardson [1866] 1952, 284.
67. Winkelstein 1995, S3.
68. Richardson [1866] 1952, 290.
69. Paneth 2004, 515.
70. Hamlin 2009, 180.
71. Freeman 1991.
72. Vinten-Johansen et al. 2003, 202.
73. Newsome 2006, 211.
74. J. Snow 1855, 20.
75. J. Snow 1855, 11.
76. J. Snow 1855, 15.
77. J. Snow 1855, 3.
78. J. Snow 1849, 29.
79. J. Snow 1855, 39.
80. J. Snow 1855, 52.
81. Rosenberg 1966, 461.
82. J. Snow 1855, 46.
83. J. Snow 1855, 42–43.
84. J. Snow 1855, 44.
85. J. Snow 1855, 44.
86. J. Snow 1855, 53.
87. J. Snow 1855, 51.
88. Gilbert 2004, 62–63.
89. J. Snow 1855, 23.
90. J. Snow 1849, 12.
91. J. Snow 1855, 56.
92. J. Snow 1855, 62–63.
93. J. Snow 1855, 64.
94. J. Snow 1855, 73.
95. J. Snow 1855, 75.
96. J. Snow 1855, 77.
97. Paneth 2004, 515.
98. J. Snow 1855, 78.
99. J. Snow 1855, 79.

100. J. Snow 1855, 86
101. J. Snow 1855, 80.
102. J. Snow 1855, 89.
103. J. Snow 1855, 109.
104. J. Snow 1855, 111.
105. J. Snow 1855, 113.
106. J. Snow 1855, 121.
107. J. Snow 1855, 121–124.
108. J. Snow 1855, 124.
109. J. Snow 1855, 32.
110. J. Snow 1855, 133–136.
111. J. Snow 1855, 136–137.
112. Wootton 2006, 195.
113. Paneth 2004, 515.
114. Vinten-Johansen et al. 2003, 342–343.
115. Ball 2009, 108.
116. Roberts 1999, 46.
117. Hempel 2013a, 1238.
118. Paneth 2004, 515.
119. S. Snow 2002, 909.
120. Koch and Denike 2009, 1247.
121. Rosenberg 1966, 456.
122. Roberts 1999, 43.
123. Hamlin 2009, 186.
124. Winkelstein 1995, S8.
125. Eyler 1973, 80–81.
126. Eyler 1973, 85.
127. J. Snow 1855, 97.
128. Eyler 1973, 84, 95, 98.
129. John Snow Archive and Research Companion, n.d., "The Cholera in Berwick Street."
130. Vinten-Johansen et al. 2003, 299.
131. Frerichs, n.d., "Reverend Henry Whitehead."
132. Vinten-Johansen et al. 2003, 299.
133. Frerichs, n.d., "Reverend Henry Whitehead."
134. Koch 2011, 215.
135. Whitehead quoted in Frerichs, n.d., "Reverend Henry Whitehead."
136. Chave 1958, 96.
137. Committee's report quoted in Frerichs, n.d., "Reverend Henry Whitehead."
138. Hempel 2013b, 1270.
139. Whitehead quoted in Frerichs, n.d., "Reverend Henry Whitehead."
140. Whitehead quoting Snow in Frerichs, n.d., "Reverend Henry Whitehead."
141. Lilienfeld 2000.
142. This quote and others to follow come from the transcripts included in Lilienfeld 2000.
143. *Lancet* quoted in Lilienfeld 2000.
144. Vinten-Johansen et al. 2003, 388–389.
145. Bynum 2013, 170.
146. Richardson [1866] 1952, 288.
147. Richardson [1866] 1952, 291.
148. Attree quoted in Hempel 2013b, 1270.
149. French quoted in Hempel 2013b, 1270.
150. Hempel 2013a, 1239.
151. Vinten-Johansen et al. 2003, 354.
152. Shapin 2006.
153. *Lancet* quoted in Vinten-Johansen et al. 2003, 394.
154. Ball 2009, 109.
155. Newsome 2006, 215.
156. Cameron and Jones 1983, 395.
157. Vinten-Johansen et al. 2003, 395.
158. Ball 2009, 109.

159. Paneth 2004, 514.
160. Freeman 1991, 293.
161. World Health Organization 2019.

Chapter 3. The Progressive Chemist
1. B. Watson 2013.
2. B. Watson 2013.
3. C. Lewis 2002, 2.
4. C. Lewis 2002, 2.
5. Wiley 1930, 217.
6. B. Watson 2013.
7. Linton 1946, 327.
8. Centers for Disease Control and Prevention 1999a.
9. Centers for Disease Control and Prevention 1999a.
10. Cole 1951, 129.
11. Cole 1951, 131–132.
12. Accum 1820, iii–iv.
13. Accum 1820, v.
14. Accum 1820, 3.
15. Accum 1820, 6, 103, 108, 268.
16. London 2014, 317–318.
17. Cole 1951, 137.
18. London 2014, 319–320.
19. Deelstra, Burns, and Walker 2014, 732.
20. Rowlinson 1982, 63.
21. Quoted in Fernandez 2018.
22. Schmid 2009, 32.
23. Fernandez 2018.
24. Blum 2018, 1.
25. Collins 1993, 101.
26. Collins 1993, 99.
27. Young 1989, 111.
28. Kurlansky 2018a, 170.
29. Kurlansky 2018a, 178–179.
30. US Food and Drug Administration 2018a.
31. Kurlansky 2018b.
32. Schmid 2009, 40.
33. Wong and Tan 2009, 235.
34. Wiley 1930, 58.
35. Wong and Tan 2009, 235.
36. Wiley 1930, 41.
37. Wiley 1930, 73.
38. Wiley 1930, 88.
39. Wiley 1930, 94–95.
40. Wiley 1930, 95.
41. Wiley 1930, 97.
42. Wiley 1930, 116.
43. Wiley 1930, 119–120.
44. Young 1989, 101.
45. Wiley 1930, 149.
46. Wong and Tan 2009, 235.
47. Wiley 1930, 151.
48. US Food and Drug Administration 2019a.
49. Wiley 1930, 160.
50. Wiley 1930, 157.
51. Wiley 1930, 157–158.
52. Young 1989, 101.
53. Wiley 1930, 154.
54. Wiley 1930, 162.
55. Wiley 1930, 165.
56. Wiley 1930, 165.
57. Wiley 1930, 166.
58. Linton 1946, 326.
59. Young 1989, 101–102.
60. D. K. Goodwin 2013.
61. Wong and Tan 2009, 235.
62. Coppin and High 1999, 34.
63. Blum 2018, 21.
64. Coppin and High 1999, 36.
65. Young 1989, 102.
66. Young 1989, 103.
67. Linton 1946, 328.
68. Coppin and High 1999, 39–40.
69. Wiley 1930, 204.
70. Young 1989, 47.
71. Wiley 1930, 205.
72. Battershall 1887, 86–87.
73. Wiley 1930, 206.

74. Quoted in D. K. Goodwin 2013, 464.
75. D. K. Goodwin 2013, 464.
76. Blum 2018, 6.
77. Coppin and High 1999, 40.
78. Wiley 1930, 184.
79. Coppin and High 1999, 44.
80. Burditt 1995, 199.
81. Wiley 1930, 190–191.
82. Wiley 1930, 223.
83. London 2014, 324.
84. Wiley 1930, 202.
85. Blum 2018, 5.
86. Linton 1946, 327.
87. Young 1989, 5.
88. Young 1989, 187–188.
89. Coppin and High 1999, 82.
90. Young 1972, 231.
91. Blum 2018, 100.
92. Young 1989, 210.
93. L. Goodwin 1999, 86.
94. Quoted in Blum 2018, 114.
95. Janssen 1981, 4.
96. L. Goodwin 1999, 88.
97. L. Goodwin 1999, 109.
98. Blum 2018, 107.
99. Young 1989, 184.
100. Lewis 2002, 1.
101. Lewis 2002, 1.
102. Lewis 2002, 1.
103. Stirling 2002, 157.
104. Lewis 2002, 1.
105. Lewis 2002, 1–2.
106. Lewis 2002, 2.
107. Wiley 1930, 219.
108. Lewis 2002, 2.
109. Lewis 2002, 2.
110. Young 1989, 155, 215.
111. Wiley 1930, 220.
112. Lewis 2002, 2.
113. Lewis 2002, 3.
114. Lewis 2002, 3.
115. US Food and Drug Administration 2019b.
116. US Food and Drug Administration 2019b.
117. US Food and Drug Administration 2019b.
118. Young 1989, 264.
119. O. Anderson 1956, 552.
120. O. Anderson 1958, 197–198.
121. Wiley 1930, 231.
122. Wiley 1930, 229.
123. Coppin and High 1999, 3.
124. Blum 2018, 152.
125. Wiley 1930, 231.
126. Linton 1946, 328.
127. Linton 1946, 328.
128. Wiley 1930, 233.
129. Wiley 1930, 236.
130. US Food and Drug Administration 2019b.
131. Wiley 1930, 239.
132. Wiley 1930, 241.
133. Coppin and High 1999, 86–87.
134. O. Anderson 1956, 563.
135. Coppin and High 1999, 159.
136. Linton 1946, 328.
137. O. Anderson 1956, 566.
138. Linton 1946, 329.
139. O. Anderson 1956, 569.
140. O. Anderson 1956, 572.
141. Kurlansky 2018a, 176, 179.
142. Kurlansky 2018a, 180–181.
143. Schmid 2009, 49.
144. Schmid 2009, 53.
145. Schmid 2009, 53–54.
146. Schmid 2009, 55.
147. Schmid 2009, 59.
148. Fernandez 2018.
149. Rankin et al. 2017, 9903.
150. Centers for Disease Control and Prevention 1999a.
151. Schmid 2009, 2–3.

152. Kurlansky 2018a, 186.
153. Blum 2018, 22.
154. Wiley 1930, 194–195.
155. Wiley 1930, 196.
156. Blum 2018, 72.
157. Wiley 1930, 197.
158. Wiley 1930, 281.
159. Blum 2018, 276.
160. *New York Times* 1964.
161. O. Anderson 1956, 568.
162. Blum 2018, 263–264.
163. Linton 1946, 329.
164. O. Anderson 1956, 550.
165. Blum 2018, 261.
166. Stirling 2002, 158.
167. Stirling 2002, 158.
168. Blum 2018, 284.
169. Stirling 2002, 158.
170. O. Anderson 1956, 573.
171. US Food and Drug Administration 2018c.
172. US Food and Drug Administration 2018b.
173. Hamburg and Sharfstein 2009, 2494.
174. US Food and Drug Administration 2018c.
175. Centers for Disease Control and Prevention 1999a.

Chapter 4. The Social Activist

1. Wald 1915, 4–6.
2. Wald 1915, 6.
3. Wald 1915, 6.
4. Wald 1915, 6.
5. Wald 1915, 8.
6. Buhler-Wilkerson 2001, 102.
7. Snyder-Grenier 2020, 4.
8. American Public Health Association, Public Health Nursing Section 2013.
9. Reverby 1993, 1662–1663.
10. Virchow quoted in Brown and Fee 2006, 2103.
11. Virchow quoted in Mackenbach 2009, 181.
12. Mackenbach 2009, 181.
13. Berridge 2016, 54.
14. Mackenbach 2009, 182.
15. Link and Phelan 1995.
16. Costa 2015, 513–514.
17. Costa 2015, 533–534.
18. Hindus 2017, ix, xv.
19. Hindus 2017, xvi.
20. Snyder-Grenier 2020, 14.
21. Hindus 2017, xvii.
22. Snyder-Grenier 2020, 12.
23. Wald 1915, 69–70.
24. Riis 1890, 105.
25. Buhler-Wilkerson 2007, 253.
26. Dingwall, Rafferty, and Webster 1988, 18.
27. Ward 2016, 26.
28. Nightingale quoted in Ward 2016, 23.
29. Ward 2016, 29.
30. Glendinning 2007.
31. Ward 2016, 31.
32. Glendinning 2007.
33. Longfellow 1857.
34. Ward 2016, 45.
35. Rosen [1958] 2015, 219–220.
36. Buhler-Wilkerson 2001, i.
37. Dingwall, Rafferty, and Webster 1988, 178.
38. Nightingale quoted in Arnott et al. 2012, 1.
39. Whelan and Buhler-Wilkerson 2011.
40. Filiaci 2016b.
41. Lagemann 1979, 1–3.
42. Daniels 1989, 11–12.
43. Lagemann 1979, 64.
44. Lagemann 1979, 65.

45. Daniels 1989, 6.
46. Lagemann 1979, 66.
47. Daniels 1989, 16.
48. Filiaci 2020.
49. Wald quoted in Feld 2008, 29.
50. Christopher, Hawkey, and Jared 2016, 197.
51. Hindus 2017, 251.
52. Filiaci 2020.
53. Buhler-Wilkerson 2001, 99.
54. Filiaci 2014.
55. Daniels 1989, 32.
56. Feld 2008, 22.
57. Wald 1915, 28.
58. Wald 1915, 2.
59. Wald 1915, 10.
60. Daniels 1989, 41.
61. Feld 2008, 32.
62. Snyder-Grenier 2020, 27.
63. Snyder-Grenier 2020, 29.
64. Lagemann 1979, 77.
65. Snyder-Grenier 2020, 26.
66. Feld 2008, 31.
67. Christopher, Hawkey, and Jared 2016, 198.
68. Snyder-Grenier 2020, 20.
69. Snyder-Grenier 2020, 20.
70. Christopher, Hawkey, and Jared 2016, 197.
71. Wald 1934, 6.
72. Buhler-Wilkerson 2001, 106.
73. Buhler-Wilkerson 2001, 106.
74. Christopher, Hawkey, and Jared 2016, 196.
75. Daniels 1989, 51–52.
76. Filiaci 2016a.
77. Feld 2008, 38.
78. Lagemann 1979, 83.
79. Feld 2008, 22.
80. Daniels 1989, 25.
81. Lagemann 1979, 79.
82. Snyder-Grenier 2020, 58.

83. Daniels 1989, 5.
84. Feld 2008, 44.
85. Daniels 1989, 13–14.
86. Feld 2008, 13.
87. Feld 2008, 30.
88. Snyder-Grenier 2020, 33.
89. Christopher, Hawkey, and Jared 2016, 202.
90. Buhler-Wilkerson 2001, 103.
91. Snyder-Grenier 2020, 34.
92. Snyder-Grenier 2020, 17.
93. Snyder-Grenier 2020, 18.
94. Wald 1915, 29.
95. Feld 2008, 59.
96. Buhler-Wilkerson 2007, 255.
97. Wald 1915, 65.
98. Buhler-Wilkerson 2001, 107.
99. Buhler-Wilkerson 2007, 255.
100. *New York Times* 1907.
101. Pittman 2019, 47.
102. Buhler-Wilkerson 2001, 110.
103. National League for Nursing 2022.
104. National League for Nursing 2022.
105. Buhler-Wilkerson 2001, 108; Christopher, Hawkey, and Jared 2016, 214.
106. Rosen [1958] 2015, 213.
107. Wald 1915, 50.
108. Rosen [1958] 2015, 214.
109. Wald 1915, 50.
110. Schumacher 2002, 247.
111. Schumacher 2002, 248.
112. San Diego County Office of Education 2013.
113. San Diego County Office of Education 2013.
114. Institute of Medicine 1997, 35.
115. Hamilton 1989, 420.
116. Hamilton 1989, 414.
117. Hamilton 1989, 421.

118. Pittman 2019, 47.
119. Hamilton 1989, 425–426.
120. Wald 1934, 286.
121. Lannon 2006, v.
122. Spreeuwenberg, Kroneman, and Paget 2018, 2561.
123. Snyder-Grenier 2020, 70.
124. Christopher, Hawkey, and Jared 2016, 212.
125. Wald 1934, 97.
126. Wald 1934, 98.
127. Stuart 2020, 108.
128. Wald 1915, 81.
129. Wald 1915, 86.
130. *New York Times* 1903.
131. Filiaci 2016c.
132. Snyder-Grenier 2020, 56.
133. Snyder-Grenier 2020, 56.
134. Wald 1915, 103.
135. Wald 1915, 108, 117, 138.
136. Christopher, Hawkey, and Jared 2016, 208.
137. Wald quoted in Oettinger 1962.
138. Roosevelt quoted in Oettinger 1962.
139. Children's Bureau 2012, 16–23.
140. Snyder-Grenier 2020, 39.
141. Wald 1934, 28.
142. Buhler-Wilkerson 2001, 112.
143. Feld 2008, 49.
144. Snyder-Grenier 2020, 40–41.
145. Buhler-Wilkerson 2001, 107.
146. Snyder-Grenier 2020, 53.
147. Wald 1915, 207.
148. Snyder-Grenier 2020, 54.
149. Buhler-Wilkerson 2001, 110.
150. Wald 1934, 14.
151. Buhler-Wilkerson 2001, 111.
152. Snyder-Grenier 2020, 72.
153. Feld 2008, 91.
154. Pittman 2019, 46.

155. Buhler-Wilkerson 1993, 1783.
156. Pittman 2019, 48.
157. Daniels 1989, 151.
158. Buhler-Wilkerson 2007, 257.
159. Pittman 2019, 47–48.
160. Christopher, Hawkey, and Jared 2016, 205.
161. Daniels 1989, 150–151.
162. Feld 2008, 120.
163. Association of Public Health Nurses 2019.
164. Association of Public Health Nurses 2019.
165. Buhler-Wilkerson 2007, 258.
166. Snyder-Grenier 2020, 1.
167. Christopher, Hawkey, and Jared 2016, 204.
168. Visiting Nurse Service of New York 2021.
169. Bosworth 2018, 248–249.
170. Centers for Disease Control and Prevention 2021a.
171. Reverby 1993, 1663.
172. Buhler-Wilkerson 1993, 1785; Pittman 2019, 51; Reverby 1993, 1663.

Chapter 5. The Social Epidemiologist

1. Baltzell 1967, xvi, xviii.
2. Anderson 1996, xiii.
3. Lindsay quoted in D. L. Lewis 1993, 179.
4. Johnson 2021a, 84.
5. Wilson et al. 1996, 78.
6. H. Gates 2007, xi.
7. Jones-Eversley and Dean 2018.
8. Krieger 2001, 693.
9. Johnson 2021a, 83.
10. K. White 2011, 290.
11. Galea and Link 2013, 846.

12. King quoted in Galarneau 2018, 5.
13. Hammonds and Reverby 2019, 1348.
14. Frankel 2000, 242.
15. Du Bois 1910, 782.
16. Frankel 2000, 242.
17. UK National Archives 2021.
18. Frankel 2000, 253.
19. Bair 2000, 281.
20. Ewbank 1987, 105.
21. Bair 2000, 289–290.
22. Frankel 2000, 276.
23. D. L. Lewis 1993, 13.
24. Du Bois 1968, 55.
25. Du Bois 1968, 55, 61.
26. D. L. Lewis 1993, 11, 79.
27. Du Bois 1968, 62.
28. D. L. Lewis 1993, 15.
29. D. L. Lewis 1993, 18.
30. Du Bois 1968, 84.
31. Du Bois 1968, 63.
32. D. L. Lewis 1993, 11.
33. Du Bois 1968, 64–65.
34. Du Bois 1968, 73, 84–85.
35. Anderson 1996, x.
36. D. L. Lewis 1993, 51.
37. Du Bois 1968, 89.
38. Du Bois 1968, 97.
39. Anderson 1996, xi.
40. Du Bois 1968, 112.
41. Du Bois 1968, 111.
42. Du Bois 1968, 115, 98.
43. D. L. Lewis 1993, 76.
44. Du Bois 1968, 99.
45. D. L. Lewis 1993, 64.
46. Du Bois 1968, 113.
47. Du Bois 1968, 115.
48. Du Bois 1968, 123, 126.
49. D. L. Lewis 1993, 80.
50. Du Bois 1968, 124.
51. Du Bois 1968, 126.
52. D. L. Lewis 1993, 100.
53. Du Bois 1968, 142.
54. D. L. Lewis 1993, 125–126.
55. Baltzell 1967, xv.
56. Du Bois 1968, 147.
57. D. L. Lewis 1993, 3–4.
58. Westbrook 2018, 200.
59. Anderson 1996, xiii.
60. Baltzell 1967, xvi.
61. Du Bois 1968, 178.
62. Du Bois 1968, 176.
63. Du Bois 1968, 183.
64. Du Bois 1968, 184.
65. D. L. Lewis 1993, 180.
66. D. L. Lewis 1993, 189.
67. Du Bois 1968, 187.
68. Bay 1998, 51.
69. Du Bois 1968, 188–189.
70. Anderson 1996, ix.
71. Du Bois 1968, 185.
72. Bobo 2007, xxv; Katz and Sugure 1998, 1.
73. Katz and Sugure 1998, 10.
74. Wilson et al. 1996, 81.
75. Du Bois [1899] 2007, 1.
76. Du Bois 1968, 188.
77. Du Bois 1968, 188.
78. Du Bois 1968, 187.
79. Johnson 2021a, 86.
80. Hunter 2015, 221.
81. Du Bois [1899] 2007, 4.
82. Jones-Eversley and Dean 2018, 233.
83. Johnson 2021a, 83.
84. Jones-Eversley and Dean 2018, 230.
85. Du Bois [1899] 2007, 109.
86. Du Bois [1899] 2007, 106.
87. Du Bois [1899] 2007, 104.
88. Du Bois [1899] 2007, 115.
89. Katz and Sugure 1998, 4.
90. Du Bois [1899] 2007, 111.

91. Du Bois [1899] 2007, 106.

92. Du Bois [1899] 2007, 104.

93. Du Bois 1906, 73.

94. Du Bois 1906, 82.

95. Du Bois 1906, 82.

96. Du Bois 1906, 90.

97. Du Bois 1906, 89.

98. Du Bois 1906, 110.

99. Du Bois [1899] 2007, 114–115.

100. Du Bois [1899] 2007, 116.

101. Wilson et al. 1996, 82.

102. Du Bois [1899] 2007, 52.

103. Du Bois [1899] 2007, 57.

104. Morris 2015, 49.

105. Du Bois [1899] 2007, 9.

106. Du Bois [1899] 2007, 12–13.

107. Du Bois [1899] 2007, 15.

108. Du Bois [1899] 2007, 16–18.

109. Du Bois [1899] 2007, 20.

110. Du Bois [1899] 2007, 19–20.

111. Du Bois [1899] 2007, 24.

112. Bobo 2000, 189.

113. Du Bois [1899] 2007, 229.

114. Du Bois [1899] 2007, 229.

115. Morris 2015, 48–49.

116. Du Bois [1899] 2007, 229–230.

117. Du Bois [1899] 2007, 234.

118. Du Bois [1899] 2007, 237.

119. Du Bois [1899] 2007, 236.

120. Du Bois [1899] 2007, 232.

121. Du Bois [1899] 2007, 235.

122. Du Bois [1899] 2007, 239.

123. Anderson 1996, xix.

124. Du Bois [1899] 2007, 234.

125. Du Bois [1899] 2007, 243.

126. Du Bois [1899] 2007, 235.

127. Du Bois 1906, 90.

128. Eaton [1899] 1996, 428.

129. Du Bois [1899] 2007, 107.

130. Du Bois [1899] 2007, 243.

131. Du Bois [1899] 2007, 246.

132. Du Bois [1899] 2007, 245.

133. Du Bois [1899] 2007, 273.

134. Du Bois [1899] 2007, 270.

135. Anderson 1996, xxv.

136. Bobo 2007, xxviii.

137. Du Bois [1899] 2007, 271.

138. Du Bois [1899] 2007, 272.

139. Bay 1998, 52.

140. Rabaka 2021, 33.

141. D. L. Lewis 1993, 210.

142. D. L. Lewis 1993, 202.

143. Baltzell 1967, xxiv.

144. Rabaka 2021, 19.

145. D. L. Lewis 1993, 207.

146. Bobo 2007, xxv.

147. Bobo 2007, xxvi.

148. Johnson 2021a, 91.

149. K. White 2011, 290.

150. Du Bois 1968, 188.

151. D. L. Lewis 1993, 194.

152. Du Bois 1968, 189.

153. Du Bois 1968, 191.

154. Du Bois 1968, 196.

155. Bobo 2007, xxix.

156. Du Bois 1968, 199.

157. Du Bois 1968, 203.

158. Du Bois 1968, 212.

159. Du Bois 1968, 212.

160. Du Bois 1968, 203.

161. Du Bois 1968, 221.

162. D. L. Lewis 1993, 4.

163. D. L. Lewis 1993, 3.

164. H. Gates 2007, xx.

165. Du Bois [1903] 2007, 1.

166. H. Gates 2007, xv.

167. Hunter 2014, 28.

168. Anderson 1996, xxx.

169. Anderson 1996, xxvi–xxviii.

170. Hunter 2014, 31.

171. Anderson 1996, xxxv.

172. Anderson 1996, ix–x.

173. Williams and Sternthal 2010, S20.

174. Williams, Lawrence, and Davis 2019, 107–108.
175. Smedley, Stith, and Nelson 2003.
176. Arias and Xu 2022, 2 (table A, with e_0 [life expectancy at birth] equal to 71.5 and 77.4).
177. Jones-Eversley and Dean 2018, 230.
178. Krieger 2001, 696.
179. Krieger 2001, 697.
180. Gee and Ford 2011, 116.
181. Galea and Link 2013, 846.
182. K. White 2011, 286.

Chapter 6. The Data Analyst

1. Peto and Beral 2010, 66–68.
2. Keating 2009, 51.
3. Peto and Beral 2010, 66.
4. Keating 2009, 52.
5. Kinlen 2005, 964.
6. Samet and Speizer 2006, 97.
7. Smith 1997, 1031.
8. Kinlen 2005, 963.
9. Keating 2009, xv.
10. Elizondo et al. 2019, 27.
11. Centers for Disease Control and Prevention 1999b.
12. Centers for Disease Control and Prevention 1999b; 2022.
13. Centers for Disease Control and Prevention 1999b; Statista Research Department 2016.
14. Centers for Disease Control and Prevention 2022.
15. Peto and Beral 2010, 66.
16. Kluger 1996, 134.
17. Hoffmann 2006, 272–273.
18. Centers for Disease Control and Prevention 1999c.
19. Wynder 1997, 688.
20. Kluger 1996, 135.
21. Kluger 1996, 135.
22. Wynder 1997, 688.
23. Keating 2009, 84.
24. American Lung Association 2021.
25. Hill, Millar, and Connelly 2003, 370.
26. Keating 2009, xv.
27. Pampel 2009, 5–7.
28. James VI of Scotland and I of England 1604.
29. Doll 1998, 90.
30. Adler 2005.
31. Loerzel 2007.
32. Loerzel 2007.
33. Doll 1998, 89.
34. Doll 1998, 91.
35. Doll 1998, 92.
36. Kluger 1996, 106.
37. Doll 1998, 111.
38. Kluger 1996, 134.
39. Thun 2005, 144.
40. Hill, Millar, and Connelly 2003, 369.
41. Doll 1998, 90.
42. Thun 2005, 144.
43. Hill, Millar, and Connelly 2003, 372.
44. Kluger 1996, 132.
45. Pampel 2009, 14–15.
46. McCormick 2018.
47. Peto and Beral 2010, 65.
48. Keating 2009, 4.
49. Peto and Beral 2010, 66; Samet and Speizer 2006, 95.
50. Darby 2003, 375.
51. Keating 2009, 9.
52. Peto and Beral 2010, 66.
53. Samet and Speizer 2006, 98.
54. Peto and Beral 2010, 66.
55. Keating 2009, 20.
56. Darby 2003, 375.

57. Peto and Beral 2010, 66.
58. Peto and Beral 2010, 67.
59. Samet and Speizer 2006, 95.
60. Peto and Beral 2010, 67.
61. Peto and Beral 2010, 67.
62. Peto and Beral 2010, 68.
63. Keating 2009, 54.
64. Peto and Beral 2010, 78.
65. Darby 2003, 375.
66. Keating 2009, 58.
67. Keating 2009, 52.
68. Kinlen 2005, 963.
69. Samet and Speizer 2006, 95.
70. Keating 2009, 58.
71. Kinlen 2005, 963.
72. Doll 1999, 290.
73. Peto and Beral 2010, 78.
74. Greene 2011, 522.
75. Peto and Beral 2010, 78.
76. Keating 2009, ix.
77. Kinlen 2005, 964.
78. Darby 2003, 377.
79. Peto and Beral 2010, 78.
80. Keating 2009, 87.
81. Keating 2009, 82.
82. Doll and Hill 1950, 741.
83. Keating 2009, 85.
84. Doll and Hill 1950, 740.
85. Keating 2009, 84.
86. Keating 2009, 88.
87. Doll and Hill 1950; Wynder and Graham 1950.
88. Kluger 1996, 133.
89. Doll and Hill 1950, 742.
90. Doll and Hill 1950, 746.
91. Doll and Hill 1950, 746.
92. Wynder and Graham 1950, 332.
93. Wynder and Graham 1950, 334.
94. Keating 2009, 108.
95. Keating 2009, 105.

96. Doll quoted in Wynder 1997, 692.
97. Keating 2009, 96.
98. Thun 2005, 144.
99. Wynder 1997, 692.
100. Wynder 1997, 693.
101. Keating 2009, 63.
102. Doll 1999, 300.
103. Hill, Millar, and Connelly 2003, 378.
104. Keating 2009, 187.
105. Doll and Hill 1950, 744–745; Doll 2002, 503–504.
106. Doll 1999, 304.
107. Peto and Beral 2010, 69.
108. Doll 2002, 500.
109. Hill 1965.
110. Hill 1965, 299.
111. Doll 2002, 500–501.
112. Doll 1999, 301.
113. Peto and Beral 2010, 69.
114. Doll and Hill 1954, 1452.
115. Peto and Beral 2010, 69.
116. Doll and Hill 1954, 1452.
117. Doll and Hill 1954, 1452.
118. Doll and Hill 1954, 1455.
119. Keating 2009, 113.
120. Mendes 2014.
121. Hammond and Horn 1954.
122. Mendes 2014.
123. Hill, Millar, and Connelly 2003, 381.
124. Doll and Hill 1964, 1400.
125. Doll and Hill 1964, 1400.
126. Doll and Hill 1964, 1401.
127. Doll and Hill 1964, 1460.
128. Doll and Hill 1964, 1466.
129. Keating 2009, 193.
130. Doll et al. 1994, 901.
131. Doll et al. 1994, 901.
132. Doll et al. 2004, 1520.
133. Doll et al. 2004, 1519.

134. US National Center for Chronic Disease Prevention and Health Promotion 2014.
135. Wynder 1997, 692.
136. Samet and Speizer 2006, 98.
137. Kinlen 2005, 964.
138. Samet and Speizer 2006, 98.
139. Keating 2009, 412.
140. Lopez 2002.
141. Medical Research Council 1957, 1524.
142. Keating 2009, 184.
143. BBC 1957.
144. Berridge 2006, 1203.
145. Berridge 2006, 1206.
146. Centers for Disease Control and Prevention 1999b
147. Centers for Disease Control and Prevention 2019.
148. Centers for Disease Control and Prevention 1999b.
149. Terry 1985, 15.
150. Centers for Disease Control and Prevention 1999b.
151. Brandt 2007, 213.
152. US National Center for Chronic Disease Prevention and Health Promotion 2014, 33.
153. Keating 2009, 439–440.
154. Peto and Beral 2010, 77.
155. Peto and Beral 2010, 77.
156. Peto and Beral 2010, 77.
157. Kinlen 2005, 964.
158. Simpson 2005, 290.
159. Smith 1997, 1031.
160. Keating 2009, 449.
161. Samet and Speizer 2006, 98.
162. Hoffmann 2006, 271.
163. Samet and Speizer 2006, 95.
164. Samet and Speizer 2006, 97.
165. Blot and Tarone 2015, 2.
166. Peto and Beral 2010, 65.
167. Elizondo et al. 2019, 27.
168. Pampel et al. 2015; Trinidad et al. 2011.
169. Wipfli and Samet 2016, 150.
170. World Health Organization 2021b.
171. Wipfli and Samet 2016, 150.
172. Wipfli and Samet 2016, 163.

Chapter 7. The International Manager

1. Maalin quoted in Global Polio Eradication Initiative 2018.
2. Kinch 2018, 52.
3. Kinch 2018, 52.
4. Kinch 2018, 53.
5. Global Polio Eradication Initiative 2018.
6. Johnson 2021a, 59.
7. Ochmann and Roser 2021.
8. Brilliant 2009.
9. Preston 2009, 14.
10. Preston 2009, 11.
11. Belongia and Naleway 2003, 88.
12. D. A. Henderson 2011, D7.
13. Preston 2009, 12.
14. G. Watson 2019.
15. Belongia and Naleway 2003, 87.
16. Geddes 2006, 152.
17. Kinch 2018, 9.
18. Geddes 2006, 153.
19. Kinch 2018, 8–9.
20. Geddes 2006, 154.
21. Riedel 2005, 22.
22. D. A. Henderson 2009, 40.
23. D. A. Henderson 2009, 41.
24. Niederhuber 2014.
25. Best, Neuhauser, and Slavin 2004, 83.
26. Stewart and Devlin 2006, 329.
27. Hager 2019.
28. Stewart and Devlin 2006, 329.

29. Riedel 2005, 22.
30. Belongia and Naleway 2003, 88.
31. Geddes 2006, 154.
32. Riedel 2005, 22.
33. Stewart and Devlin 2006, 330.
34. Best, Neuhauser, and Slavin 2004, 82.
35. Stewart and Devlin 2006, 330.
36. Riedel 2005, 23.
37. Riedel 2005, 24.
38. Stewart and Devlin 2006, 330.
39. Geddes 2006, 154.
40. Stewart and Devlin 2006, 333.
41. Johnson 2021a, 55.
42. Watson 2019.
43. Kinch 2018, 46; Watson 2019.
44. Geddes 2006, 154.
45. Belongia and Naleway 2003, 88.
46. Breman 2016, 42.
47. D. A. Henderson 2011, D8.
48. Breman 2017, 673.
49. D. A. Henderson 2009, 21.
50. Breman 2017, 673.
51. D. A. Henderson 2009, 29.
52. D. A. Henderson 2009, 22.
53. D. A. Henderson 2009, 24.
54. D. A. Henderson 2009, 23.
55. D. A. Henderson 2009, 20.
56. Johns Hopkins Bloomberg School of Public Health 2016.
57. Breman 2016, 42.
58. Johns Hopkins Bloomberg School of Public Health 2016.
59. Breman 2017, 674.
60. Branswell 2016.
61. Snyder 2016.
62. Henderson and Klepac 2013, 1.
63. D. A. Henderson 1980, 424.
64. Migiro 2016.
65. Henderson and Klepac 2013, 1.
66. Henderson and Klepac 2013, 2.
67. D. A. Henderson 2011, D8.
68. D. A. Henderson 1998, 115.
69. D. A. Henderson 2011, D8.
70. D. A. Henderson 2011, D8.
71. D. A. Henderson 1998, 115.
72. D. A. Henderson 1998, 115.
73. D. A. Henderson 2009, 77.
74. D. A. Henderson 2009, 78.
75. D. A. Henderson 2009, 105.
76. D. A. Henderson 2009, 79–80.
77. D. A. Henderson 1987a, 536.
78. D. A. Henderson 2011, D8.
79. D. A. Henderson 2009, 89.
80. D. A. Henderson 1999, S54.
81. D. A. Henderson 2009, 87.
82. D. A. Henderson 2009, 80, 86.
83. D. A. Henderson 1987b, 288.
84. D. A. Henderson 2009, 82, 85.
85. D. A. Henderson 2009, 86, 99–100, 132–133.
86. D. A. Henderson 2009, 120.
87. D. A. Henderson 2011, D9.
88. Foege 2011, 56.
89. Preston 2009, 14.
90. D. A. Henderson 2011, D8; Preston 2009, 13.
91. Henderson and Klepac 2013, 3.
92. D. A. Henderson 2011, D8.
93. Foege 2011, 49.
94. Breman 2017, 674.
95. Breman 2016, 42.
96. Foege 2011, 192.
97. D. A. Henderson 1987a, 540.
98. D. A. Henderson 2009, 169.
99. Henderson and Klepac 2013, 3.

100. Breman 2016, 42.
101. Preston 2009, 14.
102. Breman 2017, 675.
103. D. A. Henderson 1987b, 289.
104. Breman 2017, 675.
105. Breman 2017, 675.
106. D. A. Henderson 1987b, 290.
107. D. A. Henderson 2009, 137.
108. Henderson and Klepac 2013, 4.
109. D. A. Henderson 2009, 123.
110. Kinch 2018, 51.
111. Foege 2011, 46.
112. Breman 2017, 676.
113. D. A. Henderson 1998, 113.
114. D. A. Henderson 2009, 136.
115. Foege 2011, 54–56.
116. Foege 2011, 57.
117. Foege 2011, 59.
118. Foege 2011, vii.
119. Foege, Millar, and Henderson 1975, 216.
120. Breman 2017, 674.
121. D. A. Henderson 2009, 91.
122. D. A. Henderson 1972, 25.
123. Foege 2011, 77.
124. D. A. Henderson 1972, 27.
125. D. A. Henderson 1972, 28.
126. Foege 2011, 61, 66, 70–71.
127. Foege, Millar, and Henderson 1975, 218.
128. D. A. Henderson 1972, 28.
129. Foege, Millar, and Henderson 1975, 210.
130. Ogden 1987.
131. Foege, Millar, and Henderson 1975, 209.
132. Henderson and Klepac 2013, 3.
133. Quoted in Foege 2011, 73.
134. D. A. Henderson 2009, 159.
135. Foege 2011, 100.
136. Foege 2011, 164.
137. D. A. Henderson 2011, D9.
138. Foege 2011, 3.
139. Foege 2011, 111.
140. Foege 2011, 115.
141. Foege 2011, 169–172.
142. Foege 2011, 153.
143. Foege 2011, 152.
144. Foege 2011, 184.
145. D. A. Henderson 2009, 198.
146. D. A. Henderson 2009, 208.
147. D. A. Henderson 2009, 212.
148. D. A. Henderson 2009, 214, 216, 224.
149. D. A. Henderson 2009, 225.
150. D. A. Henderson 2009, 223.
151. D. A. Henderson 2009, 223–224.
152. D. A. Henderson 2009, 214.
153. D. A. Henderson 2009, 229.
154. D. A. Henderson 2011, D9.
155. D. A. Henderson 2011, D9.
156. Quoted in D. A. Henderson 1980, 422.
157. Breman 2017, 675–676.
158. Henderson and Klepac 2013, 6.
159. Henderson and Klepac 2013, 6.
160. D. A. Henderson 1980, 422.
161. Foege 2011, 183–184.
162. Johns Hopkins Bloomberg School of Public Health 2016.
163. Breman 2016, 42.
164. Johns Hopkins Bloomberg School of Public Health 2016.
165. Rimmer 2018.
166. Preston 2009, 15.
167. Belongia and Naleway 2003, 88–89.
168. Preston 2009, 17.
169. Johns Hopkins Bloomberg School of Public Health 2016.
170. Breman 2017, 676.

171. Johns Hopkins Bloomberg School of Public Health 2016.
172. Breman 2016, 42.
173. D. A. Henderson 2011, D9.
174. Okwo-Bele and Cherian 2011, D74.
175. Global Polio Eradication Initiative 2022.
176. Centers for Disease Control and Prevention 2021b; World Health Organization 2021a.
177. Centers for Disease Control and Prevention 2021b.
178. Breman 2016, 42.
179. Johnson 2021a, 51, 61.

Epilogue

1. Mackenbach 2020.
2. Mackenbach 2003.
3. Mackenbach 2020, 2.
4. Arias, Tejada-Vera, and Ahmad 2021.
5. Johnson 2021a, xxv.
6. Mackenbach 2020, 4.
7. Mackenbach 2020, 286.
8. Mackenbach 2020, 287.
9. Mackenbach 2020, 336.
10. Johnson 2021b.
11. Institute of Medicine, 1988.
12. Fairchild et al. 2010, 55.
13. Ewing 2021, 1715.
14. Ewing 2021, 1715.

REFERENCES

Accum, Friedrich. 1820. *A Treatise on Adulterations of Food and Culinary Poisons: Exhibiting the Fraudulent Sophistications of Bread, Beer, Wine, Spirituous Liquors, Tea, Coffee, Cream, Confectionery, Vinegar, Mustard, Pepper, Cheese, Olive Oil, Pickles, and Other Articles Employed in Domestic Economy, and Methods of Detecting Them.* 2nd ed. London: Longman and Associates. https://publicdomainreview.org/collection/a-treatise-on -adulteration-of-food-and-culinary-poisons-1820.

Adler, John. 2005. "Coffin Nails: The Tobacco Controversy in the 19th Century." HarpWeek Explore History. https://tobacco.harpweek .com/hubpages/CommentaryPage.asp?Commentary=Introduction.

American Lung Association. 2021. "Lung Cancer Mortality." Research and Reports. https://www.lung.org/research/trends-in-lung-disease/lung -cancer-trends-brief/lung-cancer-mortality.

American Public Health Association, Public Health Nursing Section. 2013. "The Definition and Practice of Public Health Nursing: A Statement of the Public Health Nursing Section." Washington, DC: American Public Health Association. https://www.apha.org/~/media/files/pdf/member groups/phn/nursingdefinition.ashx.

Anderson, Elijah. 1996. "Introduction to the 1996 Edition of *The Philadelphia Negro.*" In W.E.B. Du Bois, *The Philadelphia Negro: A Social Study,* ix–xxxiv. Philadelphia: University of Pennsylvania Press.

Anderson, Oscar E., Jr. 1956. "The Pure-Food Issue: A Republican Dilemma, 1906–1912." *American Historical Review* 61(3):550–573.

Anderson, Oscar E., Jr. 1958. *Health of a Nation: Harvey W. Wiley and the Fight for Pure Food.* Chicago: University of Chicago Press.

Arias, Elizabeth, Betzaida Tejada-Vera, and Farida Ahmad. 2021. "Provisional Life Expectancy Estimates for January through June, 2020." Vital Statistics Surveillance Report No. 010. National Center for Health Statistics. https://www.cdc.gov/nchs/data/vsrr/VSRR10-508.pdf.

Arias, Elizabeth, and Jiaquan Xu. 2022. "United States Life Tables, 2020." *National Vital Statistics Reports* 71(1):1–64.

Arnott, Jane, Siobhan Atherley, Joanne Kelly, and Sarah Pye. 2012. *Introduction to Community Nursing Practice*. Maidenhead, UK: McGraw-Hill Education.

Association of Public Health Nurses. 2019. "What Is a PHN?" Association of Public Health Nurses. https://www.phnurse.org/what-is-a-phn-.

Bair, Barbara. 2000. "Though Justice Sleeps: 1880–1900." In Robin D. G. Kelley and Earl Lewis, eds., *To Make Our World Anew: A History of African Americans*, 281–302. Oxford: Oxford University Press.

Ball, Laura. 2009. "Cholera and the Pump on Broad Street: The Life and Legacy of John Snow." *History Teacher* 43(1):105–119.

Baltzell, E. Digby. 1967. "Introduction to the 1967 Edition." In W.E.B. Du Bois, *The Philadelphia Negro: A Social Study*, ix–xliv. New York: Shocken Books.

Battershall, Jesse P. 1887. *Food Adulteration and Its Detection*. New York: E. & F. N. Spon.

Bay, Mia. 1998. "'The World Was Thinking Wrong about Race': *The Philadelphia Negro* and Nineteenth-Century Science." In Michael B. Katz and Thomas J. Sugure, eds., *W.E.B. DuBois, Race, and the City: "The Philadelphia Negro" and Its Legacy*, 41–60. Philadelphia: University of Pennsylvania Press.

BBC. 1957. "1957: Smoking 'Causes Lung Cancer.'" On This Day. http://news.bbc.co.uk/onthisday/hi/dates/stories/june/27/newsid_2956000/2956618.stm.

Belongia, Edward A., and Allison L. Naleway. 2003. "Smallpox Vaccine: The Good, the Bad, and the Ugly." *Clinical Medicine & Research* 1(2):87–92.

Bentham, Jeremy. 1776. *Bentham: A Fragment on Government*. Early Modern Texts. https://www.earlymoderntexts.com/assets/pdfs/bentham1776.pdf.

Berridge, Virginia. 2006. "The Policy Response to the Smoking and Lung Cancer Connection in the 1950s and 1960s." *Historical Journal* 49(4):1185–1209.

Berridge, Virginia. 2016. *Public Health: A Very Short Introduction*. Oxford: Oxford University Press.

Best, M., D. Neuhauser, and L. Slavin. 2004. "'Cotton Mather, You Dog, Dam You! I'll Inoculate You with This; with a Pox to You': Smallpox Inoculation, Boston, 1721." *Quality and Safety in Health Care* 13:82–83.

Bigelow, W. D., and Burton J. Howard. 1906. *Some Forms of Food Adulteration and Simple Methods for Their Detection*. Washington, DC: Government Printing Office. https://archive.org/stream/someformsoffooda00bigerich/someformsoffooda00bigerich_djvu.txt.

Blot, William J., and Robert E. Tarone. 2015. "Doll and Peto's Quantitative Estimates of Cancer Risks: Holding Generally True for 35 Years." *Journal of the National Cancer Institute* 107(4):1–5.

Blum, Deborah. 2018. *The Poison Squad: One Chemist's Single-Minded Crusade for Food Safety at the Turn of the Twentieth Century.* New York: Penguin Press.

Bobo, Lawrence D. 2000. "Reclaiming a Du Boisian Perspective on Racial Attitudes." *Annals, AAPSS* 568:186–202.

Bobo, Lawrence. 2007. "Introduction." In Henry Louis Gates Jr., ed., *The Philadelphia Negro: A Social Study,* xxv–xxx. Oxford: Oxford University Press.

Bosworth, Barry. 2018. "Increasing Disparities in Mortality by Socioeconomic Status." *Annual Review of Public Health* 39:237–251.

Brandt, Allan M. 2007. *The Cigarette Century: The Rise, Fall, and Deadly Persistence of the Product That Defined America.* New York: Basic Books.

Branswell, Helen. 2016. "In Death of D. A. Henderson, Credited with Eradicating Smallpox, the World Loses an Intellectual Giant." STAT. https://www.statnews.com/2016/08/21/d-a-henderson-appreciation-giant-public-health.

Breman, Joel. 2016. "Donald Ainslie Henderson (1928–2016): Epidemiologist Who Led the Effort to Eradicate Smallpox." *Nature* 538:42.

Breman, Joel. 2017. "Donald Ainslie (D. A.) Henderson, MD, MPH (1928–2016) Smallpox Eradication: Leadership and Legacy." *Journal of Infectious Diseases* 215:673–676.

Brilliant, Larry. 2009. "Critical Acclaim for Smallpox—The Death of a Disease." Frontispiece in D. A. Henderson, *Smallpox—The Death of a Disease.* Amherst, NY: Prometheus Books.

Brown, Michael. 2008. "From Foetid Air to Filth: The Cultural Transformation of British Epidemiological Thought, ca. 1780–1848." *Bulletin of the History of Medicine* 82:515–544.

Brown, Theodore M., and Elizabeth Fee. 2006. "Rudolf Carl Virchow: Medical Scientist, Social Reformer, Role Model." *American Journal of Public Health* 96(12):2102–2106.

Brundage, Anthony. 1988. *England's "Prussian Minister": Edwin Chadwick and the Politics of Government Growth, 1832–1854.* University Park: Pennsylvania State University Press.

Bryson, Bill. 2010. *At Home: A Short History of Private Life.* New York: Doubleday.

Buhler-Wilkerson, Karen. 1993. "Bringing Care to the People: Lillian Wald's Legacy to Public Health Nursing." *American Journal of Public Health* 83:1778–1786.

Buhler-Wilkerson, Karen. 2001. *No Place Like Home: A History of Nursing and Home Care in the United States*. Baltimore, MD: Johns Hopkins University Press.

Buhler-Wilkerson, Karen. 2007. "No Place Like Home: A History of Nursing and Home Care in the U.S." *Home Healthcare Nurse* 205(4):253–259.

Burditt, George M. 1995. "The History of Food Law." *Food and Drug Law Journal* 50(5):197–202.

Bynum, William. 2013. "In Retrospect: On the Mode of Communication of Cholera." *Nature* 495(March 13):169–170.

Cameron, Donald, and Ian G. Jones. 1983. "John Snow, the Broad Street Pump and Modern Epidemiology." *International Journal of Epidemiology* 12(4):393–396.

Centers for Disease Control and Prevention. 1999a. "Achievements in Public Health, 1900–1999: Safer and Healthier Foods." *MMWR* 48(40):905–913. https://www.cdc.gov/mmwr/preview/mmwrhtml /mm4840a1.htm.

Centers for Disease Control and Prevention. 1999b. "Achievements in Public Health, 1900–1999: Tobacco Use—United States, 1900–1999." *MMWR* 48(43):986–993. https://www.cdc.gov/mmwr/preview /mmwrhtml/mm4843a2.htm.

Centers for Disease Control and Prevention. 1999c. "Ernst L. Wynder, M.D." *MMWR* 48(43):987. https://www.cdc.gov/mmwr/preview /mmwrhtml/mm4843bx.htm.

Centers for Disease Control and Prevention. 2019. "A Brief History." Smoking and Tobacco Use. https://www.cdc.gov/tobacco/data _statistics/sgr/history/index.htm.

Centers for Disease Control and Prevention. 2021a. "Health Equity Considerations and Racial and Ethnic Minority Groups." COVID-19. https://www.cdc.gov/coronavirus/2019-ncov/community/health -equity/race-ethnicity.html.

Centers for Disease Control and Prevention. 2021b. "Our Progress against Polio." Global Immunization. https://www.cdc.gov/polio/progress /index.htm#:~:text=The%20annual%20number%20of%20wild, certified%20as%20eradicated%20in%202018.

Centers for Disease Control and Prevention. 2022. "Current Cigarette Smoking among Adults in the United States." Smoking and Tobacco Use. https://www.cdc.gov/tobacco/data_statistics/fact_sheets/adult _data/cig_smoking/index.htm.

Chadwick, Edwin. 1828. "An Essay on the Means of Insurance." *Westminster Review*. https://books.google.com/books?id

=5b9VAAAAcAAJ&printsec=frontcover&source=gbs_ge_summary
_r&cad=0#v=onepage&q&f=false.

Chadwick, Edwin. 1842. *Report on the Sanitary Condition of the Labouring Population of Great Britain*. London: W. Clowes and Sons. https://books.google.com/books?hl=en&lr=&id=lzK5iitgFpUC&oi=fnd&pg=PR31&dq=+ON+AN+INQUIRY+INTO+THE+SANITARY+CONDITION+LABOURING+POPULATION+OF+GREAT+BRITAIN+&ots=c5NX2dNWor&sig=PXk5Sref6bBaclbAXo_PKrP7cuk.

Chave, S.P.W. 1958. "Henry Whitehead and Cholera in Broad Street." *Medical History* 2(2): 92–108. https://www.ncbi.nlm.nih.gov/pmc/articles/PMC1034367.

Children's Bureau. 2012. "The Children's Bureau Legacy: Ensuring the Right to Childhood." US Department of Health and Human Services. https://www.childwelfare.gov/pubPDFs/cb_ebook.pdf.

Christopher, Mary Ann, Regina Hawkey, and Mary Christine Jared. 2016. "Lillian D. Wald: Pioneer of Public Health." In David Anthony Forrester, ed., *Nursing's Greatest Leaders: A History of Activism*, 195–222. New York: Springer Publishing.

Cole, R. J. 1951. "Friedrich Accum (1769–1838). A Biographical Study." *Annals of Science* 7(2):128–143.

Colgrave, James. 2002. "The McKeown Thesis: A Historical Controversy and Its Enduring Influence." *American Journal of Public Health* 95(2):725–729.

Collins, E.J.T. 1993. "Food Adulteration and Food Safety in Britain in the 19th and 20th Centuries." *Food Policy* April:95–105.

Condrau, Flurin, and Michael Worboys. 2007. "Second Opinions: Epidemics and Infections in Nineteenth-Century Britain." *Social History of Medicine* 20(1):147–158.

Conniff, Richard. 2014. "The Crank Who Made Cities Livable." Strange Behaviors. https://strangebehaviors.wordpress.com/2014/04/08/the-crank-who-made-cities-livable.

Coppin, Clayton A., and Jack High. 1999. *The Politics of Purity: Harvey Washington Wiley and the Origins of Federal Food Policy*. Ann Arbor: University of Michigan Press.

Corbett, Stephen. 1999. "Review: Public Health and Social Justice in the Age of Chadwick Britain 1800–1854." *Health Promotion International* 14(4):381–382.

Costa, Dora L. 2015. "Health and the Economy in the United States from 1750 to the Present." *Journal of Economic Literature* 53(3):503–570.

Daniels, Doris Groshen. 1989. *Always a Sister: The Feminism of Lillian D. Wald*. New York: Feminist Press.

Darby, Sarah. 2003. "A Conversation with Sir Richard Doll." *Epidemiology* 14(3):375–379.

Deelstra, H., D. Thorburn Burns, and M. J. Walker. 2014. "The Adulteration of Food, Lessons from the Past, with Reference to Butter, Margarine and Fraud." *European Food Research and Technology* 239:725–744.

Dingwall, Robert, Anne Marie Rafferty, and Charles Webster. 1988. *An Introduction to the Social History of Nursing*. London: Routledge.

Doll, Richard. 1998. "Uncovering the Effects of Smoking: Historical Perspective." *Statistical Methods in Medical Research* 7:87–117.

Doll, Richard. 1999. "Tobacco: A Medical History." *Journal of Urban Health: Bulletin of the New York Academy of Medicine* 76(3):189–313.

Doll, Richard. 2002. "Proof of Causality: Deduction from Epidemiological Observation." *Perspectives in Biology and Medicine* 45(4):499–515.

Doll, Richard, and A. Bradford Hill. 1950. "Smoking and Carcinoma of the Lung: Preliminary Report." *British Medical Journal* September 30: 739–748.

Doll, Richard, and A. Bradford Hill. 1954. "The Mortality of Doctors in Relation to Their Smoking Habits." *British Medical Journal* June 16:1451–1455.

Doll, Richard, and A. Bradford Hill. 1964. "Mortality in Relation to Smoking: Ten Years' Observations of British Doctors." *British Medical Journal* May 30:1399–1410, and June 6:1460–1467.

Doll, Richard, and Richard Peto. 1976. "Mortality in Relation to Smoking: 20 Years' Observations on Male British Doctors." *British Medical Journal* December 25:1525–1536.

Doll, Richard, Richard Peto, Jillian Boreham, and Isabelle Sutherland. 2004. "Mortality in Relation to Smoking: 50 Years' Observations on Male British Doctors." *British Medical Journal* 328:1519–1528.

Doll, Richard, Richard Peto, Keith Wheatley, Richard Gray, and Isabelle Sutherland. 1994. "Mortality in Relation to Smoking: 40 Years' Observations on Male British Doctors." *BMJ* 309:901–911. https://www.bmj.com/content/309/6959/901.

Du Bois, W.E.B. [1899] 1967. *The Philadelphia Negro: A Social Study*. Introduction by E. Digby Baltzell. New York: Shocken Books.

Du Bois, W.E.B. [1899] 1996. *The Philadelphia Negro: A Social Study*. With a new introduction by Elijah Anderson. Philadelphia: University of Pennsylvania Press.

Du Bois, W.E.B. [1899] 2007. *The Philadelphia Negro: A Social Study*. The Oxford W.E.B. Du Bois. Edited by Henry Louis Gates Jr. Introduction by Lawrence Bobo. New York: Oxford University Press.

Du Bois, W.E.B. [1903] 2007. *The Souls of Black Folk*. New York: Oxford University Press.

Du Bois, W. E. Burghardt, ed. 1906. *The Health and Physique of the Negro American: A Social Study Made under the Direction of Atlanta University by the Eleventh Atlanta Conference.* Atlanta, GA: Atlanta University Press.

Du Bois, W. E. Burghardt. 1910. "Reconstruction and Its Benefits." *American Historical Review* 15(4):781–799.

Du Bois, W.E.B. 1968. *The Autobiography of W.E.B. Du Bois: A Soliloquy on Viewing My Life from the Last Decade of Its First Century.* New York: International Publishers.

Eaton, Isabel. [1899] 1996. "Special Report on Negro Domestic Service in the Seventh Ward." In W.E.B. Du Bois, *The Philadelphia Negro: A Social Study,* 427–509. Philadelphia: University of Pennsylvania Press.

Elizondo, Enrique Loyola, Elizaveta Lebedeva, Laura Graen, Kristina Mauer-Stender, Natalia Fedkina, and Ivo Rakovac. 2019. *European Tobacco Use: Trends 2019.* Copenhagen: World Health Organization, Regional Office for Europe. https://www.euro.who.int/__data/assets/pdf_file/0009/402777/Tobacco-Trends-Report-ENG-WEB.pdf.

Ellis, Richard H. 1994. "Introduction." In Richard H. Ellis, ed., *The Case Books of Dr John Snow, Medical History, Supplement No. 14,* ix–xliii. London: Wellcome Institute for the History of Medicine.

Ewbank, Douglas C. 1987. "History of Black Mortality and Health before 1940." *Milbank Quarterly* 65(1):100–128.

Ewing, E. Thomas. 2021. "Public Health Responses to Pandemics in 1918 and 2020." *American Journal of Public Health* 111(10):1715–1717.

Eyler, John M. 1973. "William Farr on the Cholera: The Sanitarian's Disease Theory and the Statistician's Method." *Journal of the History of Medicine and Allied Sciences* 18(2):79–100.

Fairchild, Amy L., David Rosner, James Colgrove, Ronald Bayer, and Linda P. Fried. 2010. "The EXODUS of Public Health: What History Can Tell Us about the Future." *American Journal of Public Health* 100(1):54–63.

Fee, Elizabeth, and Theodore M. Brown. 2005. "The Public Health Act of 1848." *Bulletin of the World Health Organization* 83(11):866–867. http://www.who.int/bulletin/volumes/83/11/866.pdf.

Feld, Marjorie N. 2008. *Lillian Wald: A Biography.* Chapel Hill: University of North Carolina Press.

Fernandez, Daniel. 2018. "The Surprisingly Intolerant History of Milk." Smithsonian Magazine, May 11. https://www.smithsonianmag.com/history/surprisingly-intolerant-history-milk-180969056.

Filiaci, Anne M. 2014. "Juvenile Asylum." Lillian Wald—Public Health Progressive. http://www.lillianwald.com/?page_id=85.

Filiaci, Anne M. 2016a. "Building a Network of Donors and Supporters— 1893–1895." Lillian Wald—Public Health Progressive. http://www.lillianwald.com/?page_id=351.

Filiaci, Anne M. 2016b. "Lillian Wald and the Nursing Profession, 1893–1895." Lillian Wald—Public Health Progressive. http://www.lillianwald.com/?page_id=393.

Filiaci, Anne M. 2016c. "School Nurses, Section I." Lillian Wald—Public Health Progressive. http://www.lillianwald.com/?page_id=819.

Filiaci, Anne M. 2020. "Nursing School—Application and Attendance." Lillian Wald—Public Health Progressive. http://www.lillianwald.com/?page_id=1989.

Finer, S. E. 1952. *The Life and Times of Sir Edwin Chadwick*. London: Methuen.

Flinn, M. W. 1965. "Introduction." In M. W. Flinn, ed., *Report on the Sanitary Conditions of the Labouring Population of Great Britain, 1842*, 1–73. Chicago: Aldine.

Foege, William H. 2011. *House on Fire: The Fight to Eradicate Smallpox*. Berkeley: University of California Press.

Foege, William H., J. D. Millar, and D. A. Henderson. 1975. "Smallpox Eradication in West and Central Africa." *Bulletin of the World Health Organization* 52:209–222.

Foner, Eric. 1982. "Reconstruction Revisited." *Reviews in American History* 10(4):82–100.

Frankel, Noralee. 2000. "Breaking the Chains: 1760–1880. In Robin D. G. Kelley and Earl Lewis, eds., *To Make Our World Anew: A History of African Americans*, 227–280. Oxford: Oxford University Press.

Freeman, David A. 1991. "Statistical Models and Shoe Leather." *Sociological Methodology* 21:291–313.

Frerichs, Ralph R. n.d. "Broad Street Pump Outbreak." UCLA Department of Epidemiology. Accessed December 15, 2020. http://www.ph.ucla.edu/epi/snow/broadstreetpump.html.

Frerichs, Ralph R. n.d. "Index Case at 40 Broad Street." UCLA Department of Epidemiology. Accessed December 15, 2020. https://www.ph.ucla.edu/epi/snow/indexcase.html.

Frerichs, Ralph R. n.d. "Reverend Henry Whitehead." UCLA Department of Epidemiology. Accessed December 15, 2020. http://www.ph.ucla.edu/epi/Snow/whitehead.html.

Galarneau, Charlene. 2018. "Getting King's Words Right." *Journal of Health Care for the Poor and Underserved* 29(1):5–8.

Galea, Sandro, and Bruce G. Link. 2013. "Six Paths for the Future of Social Epidemiology." *American Journal of Epidemiology* 178:843–849.

Galea, Sandro, and Roger D. Vaughan. 2019. "Public Health and Marginalized Populations: A Public Health of Consequence, October 2019." *American Journal of Public Health* 109(10):1327–1328.

Gates, Bill. 2021. "Flush with Innovation: Ten Years of Reinventing the Toilet." GatesNotes. https://www.gatesnotes.com/Development/10-years-of-reinventing-the-toilet.

Gates, Henry Louis, Jr. 2007. "The Black Letters on the Sign: W.E.B. Du Bois and the Canon." In Henry Louis Gates Jr., ed., *The Philadelphia Negro*, xi–xxiv. Oxford: Oxford University Press.

Geddes, Alasdair M. 2006. "The History of Smallpox." *Clinics in Dermatology* 24:152–157.

Gee, Gilbert C., and Chandra L. Ford. 2011. "Structural Racism and Health Inequities: Old Issues, New Directions." *Du Bois Review: Social Science Research on Race* 8:115–132.

Gilbert, Pamela K. 2004. *Mapping the Victorian Social Body*. Albany: State University of New York Press.

Glendinning, Lee. 2007. "Angel of Mercy or Power-Crazed Meddler? Unseen Letters Challenge View of Pioneer Nurse." *Guardian*, September 3. https://www.theguardian.com/uk/2007/sep/03/health.health andwellbeing.

Global Polio Eradication Initiative. 2018. "Remembering Ali Maalin," September 26. https://polioeradication.org/news-post/remembering-ali -maalin.

Global Polio Eradication Initiative. 2022. "Polio Now." https://polio eradication.org. Accessed August 16, 2022.

Goodwin, Doris Kearns. 2013. *The Bully Pulpit: Theodore Roosevelt, William Howard Taft, and the Golden Age of Journalism*. New York: Simon & Schuster.

Goodwin, Lorine Swainston. 1999. *The Pure Food and Drink Crusaders, 1879–1914*. Jefferson, NC: McFarland.

Gordon, Alexander. 1897. "Dr. Thomas Southwood Smith (1788–1861)." A Web of English History. http://www.historyhome.co.uk/people/s-smith .htm.

Greene, Gayle. 2011. "Richard Doll and Alice Stewart: Reputation and the Shaping of Scientific 'Truth'" *Perspectives in Biology and Medicine* 54(4):504–531.

Hager, Thomas. 2019. "How One Daring Woman Introduced the Idea of Smallpox Inoculation to England." *Time*, March 5. https://time.com /5542895/mary-montagu-smallpox.

Halliday, Stephen. 2001. "Death and Miasma in Victorian London: An Obstinate Belief." *British Medical Journal* 323(7327):1469–1471.

Hamburg, Margaret A., and Joshua M. Sharfstein. 2009. "The FDA as a Public Health Agency." *New England Journal of Medicine* 360: 2493–2495.

Hamilton, Diane. 1989. "The Cost of Caring: The Metropolitan Life Insurance Company's Visiting Nurse Service, 1909–1953." *Bulletin of the History of Medicine* 63(3):414–434.

Hamlin, Christopher. 1996. "Edwin Chadwick, 'Mutton Medicine,' and the Fever Question." *Bulletin of the History of Medicine* 70(2): 233–265.

Hamlin, Christopher. 1998. *Public Health and Social Justice in the Age of Chadwick: Britain, 1800–1854*. Cambridge: Cambridge University Press.

Hamlin, Christopher. 2009. *Cholera: The Biography*. Oxford: Oxford University Press.

Hamlin, Christopher, and Sally Sheard. 1998. "Revolutions in Public Health: 1848, and 1998?," *BMJ* 317:587–591.

Hammond, E. Cuyler, and Daniel Horn. 1954. "The Relationship between Human Smoking Habits and Death Rates: A Follow-Up Study of 187,766 Men." *JAMA* 155(15):1316–1328.

Hammonds, Evelynn M., and Susan M. Reverby. 2019. "Toward a Historically Informed Analysis of Racial Health Disparities since 1619." *American Journal of Public Health* 109(10):1348–1349.

Hardy, Anne. 1999. "Edwin Chadwick Revisited." *Medical History* 43(2): 255–259.

Hempel, Sandra. 2007. *The Strange Case of the Broad Street Pump: John Snow and the Mystery of Cholera*. Berkeley: University of California Press.

Hempel, Sandra. 2013a. "Commentary: On the Supposed Influence of Offensive Trades on Mortality." *International Journal of Epidemiology* 42:1238–1239.

Hempel, Sandra. 2013b. "Obituary: John Snow." *Lancet* 381(April 13): 1269–1270.

Henderson, D. A. 1972. "Epidemiology in the Global Eradication of Smallpox." *International Journal of Epidemiology* 1(1):25–30.

Henderson, D. A. 1980. "Smallpox Eradication." *Public Health Reports* 95(5):422–426.

Henderson, D. A. 1987a. "Principles and Lessons from the Smallpox Eradication Programme." *Bulletin of the World Health Organization* 65(4):535–546.

Henderson, D. A. 1987b. "Smallpox Eradication: A WHO Success Story." *World Health Forum* 8:283–292.

Henderson, D. A. 1998. "Smallpox Eradication: A Cold War Victory." *World Health Bulletin* 19:113–119.

Henderson, D. A. 1999. "Lessons from the Eradication Campaigns." *Vaccine* 17:S53–S55.

Henderson, D. A. 2009. *Smallpox: The Death of a Disease*. Amherst, NY: Prometheus Books.

Henderson, D. A. 2011. "The Eradication of Smallpox—An Overview of the Past, Present, and Future." *Vaccine* 29S:D7–D9.

Henderson, D. A., and Petra Klepac. 2013. "Lessons from the Eradication of Smallpox: An Interview with D. A. Henderson." *Philosophical Transactions of the Royal Society B* 368:1–7.

Henderson, Mark. 2011. "A Clean Sweep." *Sunday Times*, May 5. https://www.thetimes.co.uk/article/a-clean-sweep-o8mqrrrm7og.

Hill, A. Bradford. 1965. "The Environment and Disease: Association or Causation?," *Proceedings of the Royal Society of Medicine* 58:295-300.

Hill, Gerry, Wayne Millar, and James Connelly. 2003. "'The Great Debate': Smoking, Lung Cancer, and Cancer Epidemiology." *Canadian Bulletin of Medical History* 20(2):367-386.

Hindus, Milton. 2017. "Introduction." In Milton Hindus, ed., *The Jewish East Side 1881-1924*, xv-xxxii. London: Routledge.

Hoffmann, Ilse. 2006. "Biosketch of Ernst Ludwig Wynder." *Preventive Medicine* 43:271-273.

Hunter, Marcus Anthony. 2014. "Black Philly after *The Philadelphia Negro*." *Contexts* 13(1):26-31.

Hunter, Marcus Anthony. 2015. "W.E.B. Du Bois and Black Heterogeneity: How *The Philadelphia Negro* Shaped American Sociology." *American Sociologist* 46:219-233.

Institute of Medicine. 1988. "Summary and Recommendations." In *The Future of Public Health*. Washington, DC: National Academies Press. https://www.ncbi.nlm.nih.gov/books/NBK218215/#ddd00012.

Institute of Medicine. 1997. *Schools & Health: Our Nation's Investment*. Washington, DC: National Academies Press. http://www.nap.edu/openbook.php?record_id=5153&page=35.

Jackson, Lee. 2014. *Dirty Old London: The Victorian Fight against Filth*. New Haven, CT: Yale University Press.

James VI of Scotland and I of England (king). 1604. "A Counterblast to Tobacco." Ex-Classics Web Site. https://www.exclassics.com/blasts/tobintro.htm.

Janssen, Wallace F. 1981. "The Story of the Laws behind the Labels." *FDA Consumer Magazine* June:1-16.

Janssen, Wallace F. 1987. "Inside the Poison Squad: How Food Additive Regulation Began." *Association of Food and Drug Officials Quarterly Bulletin* 51(2):68-72.

Johns Hopkins Bloomberg School of Public Health. 2016. "Donald Ainslie Henderson MD, MPH '60: 1928-2016." Heroes of Public Health. https://publichealth.jhu.edu/about/history/heroes-of-public-health/donald-a-henderson.

John Snow Archive and Research Companion. n.d. "The Cholera of Berwick Street." Michigan State University. Accessed November 28, 2020. https://johnsnow.matrix.msu.edu/work.php?id=15-78-7C.

John Snow Archive and Research Companion. n.d. "John Snow's Published Works." Michigan State University. Accessed November 28, 2020. https://johnsnow.matrix.msu.edu/publications.php.

John Snow Archive and Research Companion. n.d. "On Asphyxia, and on the Resuscitation of Still-Born Children." Michigan State University. Accessed November 28, 2020. https://johnsnow.matrix.msu.edu/work .php?id=15-78-D.

John Snow Society. 2020. "Welcome to the John Snow Society." www .johnsnowsociety.org.

Johnson, Steven. 2006. *The Ghost Map: The Story of London's Most Terrifying Epidemic—and How It Changed Science, Cities, and the Modern World.* New York: Riverhead Books.

Johnson, Steven. 2021a. *Extra Life: A Short History of Living Longer.* New York: Riverhead Books.

Johnson, Steven. 2021b. "How Humanity Gave Itself an Extra Life." *New York Times Magazine,* April 27. https://www.nytimes.com/2021/04/27 /magazine/global-life-span.html.

Jones-Eversley, Sharon D., and Lorraine T. Dean. 2018. "After 121 Years, It's Time to Recognize W.E.B. Du Bois as a Founding Father of Social Epidemiology." *Journal of Negro Education* 87(3):230-245.

Katz, Michael B., and Thomas J. Sugure. 1998. "Introduction: The Context of *The Philadelphia Negro.*" In Michael B. Katz and Thomas J. Sugure, eds., *W.E.B. DuBois, Race, and the City: The Philadelphia Negro and Its Legacy,* 1-38. Philadelphia: University of Pennsylvania Press.

Keating, Conrad. 2009. *Smoking Kills: The Revolutionary Life of Richard Doll.* Oxford: Signal Books.

Kinch, Michael. 2018. *Between Hope and Fear: A History of Vaccines and Human Immunity.* New York: Pegasus Books.

Kinlen, Leo. 2005. "Sir Richard Doll, Epidemiologist—A Personal Reminiscence with a Selected Bibliography." *British Journal of Cancer* 93:963-966.

Kluger, Richard. 1996. *Ashes to Ashes: America's Hundred-Year Cigarette War, the Public Health, and the Unabashed Triumph of Philip Morris.* New York: Alfred A. Knopf.

Koch, Tom. 2011. *Disease Maps: Epidemics on the Ground.* Chicago: University of Chicago Press.

Koch, Tom, and Kenneth Denike. 2009. "Crediting His Critics' Concerns: Remaking John Snow's Map of Broad Street Cholera, 1854." *Social Science & Medicine* 69:1246-1251.

Krieger, N. 2001. "A Glossary for Social Epidemiology." *Journal of Epidemiology & Community Health* 55:693-700.

Kurlansky, Mark. 2018a. *Milk! A 10,000-Year Food Fracas.* New York: Bloomsbury.

Kurlansky, Mark. 2018b. "Why We've Been Fighting about Milk for 10,000 Years." *Time,* May 27. https://time.com/5244870/milk-history -mark-kurlansky.

Lagemann, Ellen Condliffe. 1979. *A Generation of Women: Education in the Lives of Progressive Reformers.* Cambridge, MA: Harvard University Press.

Lannon, Thomas G. 2006. "Lillian Wald Papers: 1889–1957." New York Public Library. https://www.nypl.org/sites/default/files/blog _attachments/wald.pdf.

Lewis, Carol. 2002. "The 'Poison Squad' and the Advent of Food and Drug Regulation." *U.S. Food and Drug Administration Consumer Magazine* November–December:1–15.

Lewis, David Levering. 1993. *W.E.B. Du Bois: Biography of a Race, 1868– 1919.* New York: Holt.

Lilienfeld, David E. 2000. "John Snow: The First Hired Gun?" *American Journal of Epidemiology* 152(1): 4–9. https://academic.oup.com/aje /article/152/1/4/139165.

Link, Bruce G., and Jo Phelan. 1995. "Social Conditions as Fundamental Causes of Disease." *Journal of Health and Social Behavior* Extra Issue:80–94.

Linton, Fred B. 1946. "Its Distinguished Administrators." *Food Drug Cosmetic Law Quarterly* September:326–333.

Listios, Socrates. 2003. "Charles Dickens and the Movement for Sanitary Reform." *Perspectives in Biology and Medicine* 46(2):183–199.

LiveScience Staff. 2009. "Ganges Delta: Gorgeous, Wild, and Deadly." *LiveScience*, August 7. https://www.livescience.com/5608-ganges-delta -gorgeous-wild-deadly.html.

Loerzel, Robert. 2007. "The Smoking Gun." *Chicago* magazine, December 31. https://www.chicagomag.com/Chicago-Magazine/January -2008/The-Smoking-Gun.

London, Jillian. 2014. "Tragedy, Transformation, and Triumph: Comparing the Factors and Forces That Led to the Adoption of the 1860 Adulteration Act in England and the 1906 Pure Food and Drug Act in the United States." *Food and Drug Law Journal* 69(2):315–342.

Longfellow, Henry Wadsworth. 1857. "Santa Filomena." *Atlantic*, November. *The Atlantic* Ideas Tour. https://www.theatlantic.com/ideastour /archive/longfellow.html.

Lopez, Steve. 2002. "Big Tobacco Is Cursing the Day This Expert Witness Took the Oath." *Los Angeles Times*, August 25. https://www.latimes.com /archives/la-xpm-2002-aug-25-me-lopez25-story.html.

Mackenbach, Johan. 2003. Interview in Dissecting Room / Lifeline. *Lancet* 361(9356):538.

Mackenbach, Johan. 2009. "Politics Is Nothing but Medicine at a Larger Scale: Reflections on Public Health's Biggest Idea." *Journal of Epidemiology & Community Health* 63:181–184.

Mackenbach, Johan. 2020. *A History of Population Health: Rise and Fall of Disease in Europe.* Leiden: Brill.

Marston, Maurice. 1925. *Sir Edwin Chadwick.* London: Lenard Parsons.

McCormick, Kevin. 2018. "17 Vintage Lucky Strike Ads." Pretty Sweet. https://prettysweet.com/lucky-strike-ads-smoking-diet.

McKeown, Thomas. 1976a. *The Modern Rise of Population.* New York: Academic Press.

McKeown, Thomas. 1976b. *The Role of Medicine: Dream, Mirage, or Nemesis?* London: Nufflield Provincial Hospitals Trust.

McKeown, Thomas, and R. G. Brown. 1955. "Medical Evidence Related to English Population Changes in the Eighteenth Century." *Population Studies* 9(2):119–141.

McKeown, Thomas, and R. G. Record. 1962. "Reasons for the Decline of Mortality in England and Wales during the Nineteenth Century." *Population Studies* 16(2):94–122.

McNeil, Donald G., Jr. 2019. "The Ganges Brims with Dangerous Bacteria." *New York Times,* December 23. https://www.nytimes.com/2019/12/23/health/ganges-drug-resistant-bacteria.html.

Medical Research Council. 1957. "Tobacco Smoking and Cancer of the Lung: Statement by the Medical Research Council." *British Medical Journal* June 29:1523–1524.

Mendes, Elizabeth. 2014. "The Study That Helped Spur the U.S. Stop-Smoking Movement." American Cancer Society. https://www.cancer.org/latest-news/the-study-that-helped-spur-the-us-stop-smoking-movement.html.

Migiro, Katy. 2016. "Timeline: The Long Road to Malaria Eradication." Reuters. https://www.reuters.com/article/us-africa-malaria-events-timeline/timeline-the-long-road-to-malaria-eradication-idUSKCN0YU0ER.

Morris, Aldon D. 2015. *The Scholar Denied: W.E.B. Du Bois and the Birth of Modern Sociology.* Oakland: University of California Press.

National League for Nursing. 2022. "Historical Timeline." National League for Nursing. https://www.nln.org/docs/default-source/uploadedfiles/default-document-library/nln-timeline-june-2020.pdf?sfvrsn=16f6a70d_0.

Newsome, S.W.B. 2006. "Pioneers in Infection Control: John Snow, Henry Whitehead, the Broad Street Pump, and the Beginnings of Geographical Epidemiology." *Journal of Hospital Infection* 64:210–216.

New York Times. 1903. "Seward Park Is Opened: Mayor Low Speaks to Vast Crowd Gathered in the Rain." *New York Times,* October 18.

New York Times. 1907. "Unique Settlement on Henry Street: In This District the Sick Are Given All Necessary Care and Proper Nursing at Their Homes Instead of Going to Hospital." *New York Times,* July 21.

New York Times. 1964. "Mrs. H. W. Wiley, Suffragette, Dies: Aided Husband in Fight for Pure Food and Drug Law." *New York Times* Archive, January 4. https://www.nytimes.com/1964/01/07/archives/mrs-h-w-wiley -suffragette-dies-aided-husband-in-fight-for-pure-food.html.

Niederhuber, Matthew. 2014. "The Fight over Inoculation during the 1721 Boston Smallpox Epidemic." Harvard University Graduate School of Arts and Sciences. https://sitn.hms.harvard.edu/flash/special-edition -on-infectious-disease/2014/the-fight-over-inoculation-during-the-1721 -boston-smallpox-epidemic.

Ochmann, Sophie, and Max Roser. 2021. "Smallpox." Our World in Data. https://ourworldindata.org/smallpox.

Oettinger, Katherine B. 1962. "It's Your Children's Bureau." Social Security. The Children's Bureau. https://www.ssa.gov/history/childb2.html.

Ogden, Horace G. 1987. *CDC and the Smallpox Crusade*. Washington, DC: US Government Printing Office.

Okwo-Bele, Jean Marie, and Thomas Cherian. 2011. "The Expanded Program on Immunization: A Lasting Legacy of Smallpox Eradication." *Vaccine* 29S:D74–D79.

Pampel, Fred C. 2009. *Tobacco Industry and Smoking*. 2nd ed. New York: Facts on File.

Pampel, Fred, Stephane Legleye, Céline Goffette, Daniela Pointek, Ludwig Kraus, and Myriam Khlat. 2015. "Cohort Changes in Educational Disparities in Smoking: France, Germany and the United States." *Social Science & Medicine* 127:41–50.

Paneth, Nigel. 2004. "Assessing the Contributions of John Snow to Epidemiology: 150 Years after Removal of the Broad Street Pump Handle." *Epidemiology* 15(5): 514–516.

Peto, Richard, and Valerie Beral. 2010. "Sir Richard Doll: 28 October 1912– 24 July 2005." *Biographical Memoirs of the Fellows of the Royal Society* 56:63–83.

Pflaumer, Peter. 2015. "Estimation of the Roman Life Expectancy Using Ulpian's Table." *JMS Proceedings, Social Statistics Section*. https://core.ac .uk/download/pdf/46916547.pdf.

Phillips, David. 2003. "Three 'Moral Entrepreneurs' and the Creation of a 'Criminal Class' in England, c. 1790s–1840s." *Crime, History & Societies* 7(1):79–107.

Pittman, Patricia. 2019. "Rising to the Challenge: Re-embracing the Wald Model of Nursing." *American Journal of Nursing* 119(7):46–52.

Pollitzer, R. 1954. "Cholera Studies." *Bulletin of the World Health Organization* 10:421–461.

Poor Law Commission. 1834. *Poor Law Commission's Report of 1834*. London: His Majesty's Stationary Office. https://oll.libertyfund.org/title/chadwick -poor-law-commissioners-report-of-1834.

Porter, Dorothy. 1998. *Health, Civilization, and the State*. London: Routledge.

Poynter, F.N.L. 1962. "Thomas Southwood Smith—the Man (1788–1861). *Proceedings of the Royal Society of Medicine* 55:381–392.

Preston, Richard. 2009. "Foreword." In D. A. Henderson, *Smallpox: The Death of a Disease*, 11–18. Amherst NY: Prometheus Books.

Queijo, Jon. 2010. *Breakthrough! How the 10 Greatest Discoveries in Medicine Saved Millions and Changed Our View of the World*. Upper Saddle River, NJ: FT Press Science.

Rabaka, Reiland. 2021. *Du Bois: A Critical Introduction*. Cambridge: Polity Press.

Rankin, S. A., R. L. Bradley, G. Miller, and K. B. Mildenhall. 2017. "A 100-Year Review: A Century of Dairy Processing Advancements— Pasteurization, Cleaning and Sanitation, and Sanitary Equipment Design." *Journal of Dairy Science* 100:9903–9915.

Reverby, Susan M. 1993. "From Lillian Wald to Hillary Rodham Clinton: What Will Happen to Public Health Nursing?" *American Journal of Public Health* 83(12):1662–1663.

Richardson, Benjamin Ward. [1866] 1952. "John Snow, M.D., a Representative of Medical Science and Art of the Victorian Era." In *Asclepiad*, reprinted in *British Journal of Anaesthesia* 24:267–291.

Riedel, Stefan. 2005. "Edward Jenner and the History of Smallpox and Vaccination." *BUMC Proceedings* 18:21–25.

Riis, Jacob A. 1890. *How the Other Half Lives: Studies among the Tenements of New York*. New York: C. Scribner's Sons.

Rimmer, Monica. 2018. "How Smallpox Claimed Its Final Victim." BBC News, August 10. https://www.bbc.com/news/uk-england-birmingham -45101091.

Roberts, Shirley. 1999. "John Snow (1813–1858) and Benjamin Ward Richardson (1828–1896): A Notable Friendship." *Journal of Medical Biography* 7:42–49.

Rosen, George. [1958] 2015. *A History of Public Health*. Rev. exp. ed. Baltimore, MD: Johns Hopkins University Press.

Rosenberg, Charles E. 1966. "Cholera in Nineteenth-Century Europe: A Tool for Social and Economic Analysis." *Comparative Studies in Society and History* 8(4):452–463.

Rowlinson, P. J. 1982. "Food Adulteration: Its Control in 19th Century Britain." *Interdisciplinary Science Reviews* 7(1):63–72.

Samet, Jonathan M., and Frank E. Speizer. 2006. "Sir Richard Doll, 1912–2005." *American Journal of Epidemiology* 164(1):95–100.

San Diego County Office of Education. 2013. "A Brief History of School Nursing." https://www.sdcoe.net/student-services/student-support /Documents/Nursing/school-nursing-history.pdf.

Schmid, Ron. 2009. *The Untold Story of Milk, Revised and Updated: The History, Politics and Science of Nature's Perfect Food; Raw Milk from Pasture-Fed Cows*. Washington, DC: New Trends Publishing.

Schumacher, Casey. 2002. "Lina Rogers: A Pioneer in School Nursing." *Journal of School Nursing* 18(5):247–249.

Shapin, Steven. 2006. "Sick City: Maps and Mortality in the Time of Cholera." *New Yorker*, November 6. https://www.newyorker.com /magazine/2006/11/06/sick-city.

Simpson, D. 2005. "Sir Richard Doll, 1912–2005." *Tobacco Control* 14:289–290.

Smedley, B. D., A. Y. Stith, and A. R. Nelson. 2003. *Unequal Treatment: Confronting Racial and Ethnic Disparities in Health Care*. Washington, DC: National Academies Press. https://www.nap.edu/catalog/10260 /unequal-treatment-confronting-racial-and-ethnic-disparities-in -health-care.

Smith, Richard. 1997. "Richard Doll at 85." *British Medical Journal* October 25:1031.

Snow, John. 1849. *On the Mode of Communication of Cholera*. London: John Churchill.

Snow, John. 1855. *On the Mode of Communication of Cholera*. 2nd ed. London: John Churchill.

Snow, Stephanie J. 2000a. "John Snow MD (1813–1858): Part I, A Yorkshire Childhood and Family Life." *Journal of Medical Biography* 8:27–31.

Snow, Stephanie J. 2000b. "John Snow MD (1813–1858): Part II, Becoming a Doctor—His Medical Training and Early Years of Practice." *Journal of Medical Biography* 8:71–77.

Snow, Stephanie J. 2002. "Commentary: Sutherland, Snow and Water; The Transmission of Cholera in the Nineteenth Century." *International Journal of Epidemiology* 31:908–911.

Snow, Stephanie J. 2008. "John Snow: The Making of a Hero?" *Lancet* 372:22–23.

Snyder, Alison. 2016. "Donald A. Henderson." *Lancet* 388:1050. https:// www.thelancet.com/journals/lancet/article/PIIS0140-6736(16)31548-3 /fulltext?rss=yes.

Snyder-Grenier, Ellen M. 2020. *The House on Henry Street: The Enduring Life of a Lower East Side Settlement*. New York: New York University Press.

Spreeuwenberg, P., M. Kroneman, and J. Paget. 2018. "Reassessing the Global Mortality Burden of the 1918 Influenza Pandemic." *American Journal of Epidemiology* 187(12):2561–2567.

Statista Research Department. 2016. "Per Capita Cigarette Consumption in the United States from 1900 to 2015." Statista. https://www.statista.com /statistics/261576/cigarette-consumption-per-adult-in-the-us.

Stewart, Alexandra J., and Phillip M. Devlin. 2006. "The History of the Smallpox Vaccine." *Journal of Infection* 52:329–334.

Stirling, Dale A. 2002. "Profiles in Toxicology: Harvey W. Wiley." *Toxicological Sciences* 67:157–158.

Stuart, Paul H. 2020. "Lillian Wald Reports on Organizing to Combat the 1918 Influenza Pandemic in New York City." *Journal of Community Practice* 28(2):100–111.

Szreter, Simon. 1988. "The Importance of Social Intervention in Britain's Mortality Decline c. 1850–1914: A Re-interpretation of the Role of Public Health." *Social History of Medicine* 1(1):1–38.

Terry, Luther L. 1985. "The Surgeon General's First Report on Smoking and Health." In Alan Blum, ed., *The Cigarette Underworld: A Front Line Report on the War against Your Lungs*, 14–24. Secaucus, NJ: Lyle Stuart.

Teutsch, Steven M., and Jonathan E. Fielding. 2013. "Rediscovering the Core of Public Health." *Annual Review of Public Health* 34:287–299.

Thun, Michael J. 2005. "When Truth Is Unwelcome: The First Reports on Smoking and Lung Cancer." *Bulletin of the World Health Organization* 83(2):144–145.

Trinidad, Dennis R., Eliseo J. Perez-Stable, Martha M. White, Sherry L. Emery, and Karen Messer. 2011. "A Nationwide Analysis of US Racial/Ethnic Disparities in Smoking Behaviors, Smoking Cessation, and Cessation-Related Factors." *American Journal of Public Health* 101(4):699–706.

United Kingdom. National Archives. 2021. "Great Plague of 1665–1666." http://www.nationalarchives.gov.uk/education/resources/great-plague/#external-links.

United States. National Archives. 2022. "The Freedmen's Bureau." African American Heritage. https://www.archives.gov/research/african-americans/freedmens-bureau.

US Food and Drug Administration. 2018a. "The Dangers of Raw Milk: Unpasteurized Milk Can Pose a Serious Health Risk." Buy, Store, and Serve Safe Food. https://www.fda.gov/food/buy-store-serve-safe-food/dangers-raw-milk-unpasteurized-milk-can-pose-serious-health-risk.

US Food and Drug Administration. 2018b. "FDA Mission." What We Do. https://www.fda.gov/about-fda/what-we-do.

US Food and Drug Administration. 2018c. "Milestones in U.S. Food and Drug Law History." https://www.fda.gov/about-fda/fdas-evolving-regulatory-powers/milestones-us-food-and-drug-law-history.

US Food and Drug Administration. 2019a. Tweet, February 3. https://twitter.com/us_fda/status/1092196031557558273.

US Food and Drug Administration. 2019b. "Part I: The 1906 Food and Drug Act and Its Enforcement." The History of FDA's Fight for Con-

sumer Protection and Public Health. https://www.fda.gov/about-fda
/changes-science-law-and-regulatory-authorities/part-i-1906-food-and
-drugs-act-and-its-enforcement.

US National Center for Chronic Disease Prevention and Health Promotion.
Office on Smoking and Health. 2014. *The Health Consequences of
Smoking—50 Years of Progress: A Report of the Surgeon General*. Atlanta,
GA: Centers for Disease Control and Prevention.

Vinten-Johansen, Peter, Howard Brody, Nigel Paneth, Stephen Rachman,
Michael Rip, and David Zuck. 2003. *Cholera, Chloroform, and the
Science of Medicine: A Life of John Snow*. Oxford: Oxford University
Press.

Visiting Nurse Service of New York. 2021. "About Us." https://www.vnsny
.org/who-we-are/about-us.

Wald, Lillian. 1915. *The House on Henry Street*. New York: Henry Holt.

Wald, Lillian. 1934. *Windows on Henry Street*. Boston: Little Brown.

Ward, Francis. 2016. "Florence Nightingale: Where Most Work Is Wanted."
In David Anthony Forrester, ed., *Nursing's Greatest Leaders: A History of
Activism*, 21–54. New York: Springer.

Watson, Bruce. 2013. "The Poison Squad: An Incredible History." *Esquire*,
June 27. https://www.esquire.com/food-drink/food/a23169/poison
-squad.

Watson, Grieg. 2019. "The Anti-Vaccination Movement That Gripped
Victorian England." BBC News, December 28. https://www.bbc.com
/news/uk-england-leicestershire-50713991.

Westbrook, Randall O. 2018. "Dr. W.E.B. Du Bois and the Enduring
Significance of *The Philadelphia Negro*." *Journal of Negro Education*
87(3):200–201.

Whelan, Jean C., and Karen Buhler-Wilkerson. 2011. "Nursing through
Time: 1870–1899." Nursing, History, and Health Care. https://www
.nursing.upenn.edu/nhhc/nursing-through-time/1870-1899.

White, Kellee. 2011. "The Sustaining Relevance of W.E.B. Du Bois to
Health Disparities Research." *Du Bois Review* 8(1):285–293.

White, Matthew. 2009. "The Rise of Cities in the 18th Century." British
Library. http://www.bl.uk/georgian-britain/articles/the-rise-of-cities
-in-the-18th-century.

Wiley, Harvey W. 1930. *An Autobiography*. Indianapolis, IN: Bobbs-Merrill.

Williams, David R., Jourdyn A. Lawrence, and Brigette A. Davis. 2019.
"Racism and Health: Evidence and Needed Research." *Annual Review of
Public Health* 40:105–125.

Williams, David R., and Michelle Sternthal. 2010. "Understanding Racial-
Ethnic Disparities in Health: Sociological Contributions." *Journal of
Health and Social Behavior* 51(suppl.):S15–S27.

Wilson, William Julius, Gerald Early, David Levering Lewis, Elijah Anderson, James E. Blackwell, Ronald Walters, and Chuck Stone. 1996. "Du Bois' *The Philadelphia Negro*: 100 Years Later." *Journal of Blacks in Higher Education* 11(Spring):78–84.

Winkelstein, Warren, Jr. 1995. "A New Perspective on John Snow's Communicable Disease Theory." *American Journal of Epidemiology* 142(9 suppl.): S3–S9.

Winslow, C.E.A. 1920. "The Untilled Fields of Public Health." *Science* 51:23–33.

Wipfli, Heather, and Jonathan M. Samet. 2016. "One Hundred Years in the Making: The Global Tobacco Epidemic." *Annual Review of Public Health* 37:149–166.

Wong, V., and S. Y. Tan. 2009. "Harvey Washington Wiley (1844–1930): Champion of the Pure Food and Drugs Act." *Singapore Medical Journal* 50(3):235–236.

Wootton, David. 2006. *Bad Medicine: Doctors Doing Harm since Hippocrates*. New York: Oxford University Press.

World Health Organization. 2019. "Cholera." https://www.who.int/news-room/fact-sheets/detail/cholera.

World Health Organization. 2021a. "Countries Reaffirm Commitment to Ending Polio at Launch of New Eradication Strategy." https://www.who.int/news/item/10-06-2021-countries-reaffirm-commitment-to-ending-polio-at-launch-of-new-eradication-strategy.

World Health Organization. 2021b. "Key Facts." Tobacco. https://www.who.int/news-room/fact-sheets/detail/tobacco.

World Health Organization. 2022. "Sanitation." https://www.who.int/news-room/fact-sheets/detail/sanitation#:~:text=Poor%20sanitation%20is%20linked%20to,assault%2C%20and%20lost%20educational%20opportunities.

Wynder, Ernest L. 1997. "Tobacco as a Cause of Lung Cancer: Some Reflections." *American Journal of Epidemiology* 146(9):687–694.

Wynder, Ernest L., and Evarts A. Graham. 1950. "Tobacco Smoking as a Possible Etiologic Factor in Bronchiogenic Carcinoma: A Study of Six Hundred and Eighty-Four Proved Cases." *JAMA* 143(4):329–336.

Young, James Harvey. 1972. *The Toadstool Millionaires: A Social History of Patent Medicines in America before Federal Regulation*. Princeton, NJ: Princeton University Press.

Young, James Harvey. 1989. *Pure Food: Securing the Federal Food and Drugs Act of 1906*. Princeton, NJ: Princeton University Press.

Zuberi, Tukufo. 2004. "W.E.B. Du Bois's Sociology: *The Philadelphia Negro* and Social Science." *Annals, AAPSS* 595:146–156.

INDEX

Accum, Friedrich, 89–92, 103
Addams, Jane, 144
Adulteration Act (Great Britain, 1860), 92
African Americans: Black Codes, 173; common interests, 196; discrimination against, 191–194, 196–199, 202; diversity of, 188–189; electoral success, 172; employment restrictions on, 192–193; health and mortality, 175–176, 185–188, 195, 200, 202; Jim Crow, 174–175, 199; lynching, 160, 174, 176; migration from South, 188–189, 191; migration to North, 175; Philadelphia, history in, 189–191; racism, 170, 183, 185, 189, 199–200, 202; Reconstruction, hopes for, 172–173; segregation, 174–176, 178–180, 199, 202; sharecroppers, 173; slavery, 171–172, 190, 192; stereotyping of, 183, 188, 193; voting rights, 175; white prejudice, 192–194; women, 194–195
American Cancer Society, smoking and lung cancer study, 228–229
American Civil Liberties Union, 155
Anderson, Elijah, 201
anesthesiology, 55, 57
Anti-Cigarette League, 212
Atlanta University, 198–199
Autobiography, An (Wiley, 1930), 122

Bazalgette, Sir Joseph William, 80
Bentham, Jeremy, 3, 16–17, 22
Berlin, Irving (Israel Beilin), 133
Berridge, Virginia, 3
Bill and Melinda Gates Foundation: polio initiative, 271, 273; toilet challenge sponsorship, 41

Black Codes, 173
Blum, Deborah, 93–94
Bragg, Nana, 250
Brazil, 264
Brewster, Mary, 127, 142–144
British Medical Association, 228
British Medical Journal, 207, 221, 236
Broad Street pump, 60–63, 75–76
Brown, George Rothwell, 86
Brown v. Board of Education, 175
Brundage, Anthony, 21
Bryson, Bill, 10
Budd, William, 73
Buhler-Wilkerson, Karen, 150
Bulletin 13 on Foods and Food Adulteration (US Department of Agriculture, 1887–1907), 103, 105, 107

cancer, 206, 210. *See also* lung cancer
Candau, Marcelino, 253, 256
case-control tobacco study, 219–222; criticisms of, 225; government response to, 223; limitations, 227–228; reactions of scientists to, 224; results, 220–222; sample used, 220; strengths, 219, 225–226; tobacco company response to, 223
causality, tobacco and lung cancer, 222; debate over, 223–227, 229; new understanding of, 226; probabilities, implications of, 224–225; standard of proof used, 224
Centers for Disease Control and Prevention (CDC), 124, 271–273; Epidemic Intelligence Service, 250; smallpox eradication efforts, 260–262, 265; surveillance importance, 251–252